高等院校药学类专业双语实验教材

药物化学双语实验

主　编　温新民　綦慧敏

副主编　李　伟　管　华　王其宝　刘冬梅

编　委（以姓氏笔画为序）

王其宝（济宁医学院）　　　　刘冬梅（潍坊医学院）

刘潇潇（潍坊医学院）　　　　闫玉刚（济宁医学院）

孙延龙（潍坊医学院）　　　　李　伟（济宁医学院）

贾海永（潍坊医学院）　　　　温新民（济宁医学院）

曾现忠（潍坊医学院）　　　　綦慧敏（潍坊医学院）

管　华（济宁医学院）

中国健康传媒集团

中国医药科技出版社

内 容 提 要

本教材是"高等院校药学类专业双语实验教材"中的一本。本套教材由济宁医学院联合潍坊医学院共同编写。为适应医药行业国际化对药学类人才的需求，结合目前大学生英语水平普遍较高的特点，本套教材采用中英文双语编写。本教材共包括药物化学实验基本知识、药物合成实验、附录三个部分，其中第二部分包括 11 个实验。

本教材适合高等药学院校药学类专业使用。

图书在版编目（CIP）数据

药物化学双语实验 / 温新民，綦慧敏主编. —北京：中国医药科技出版社，2019.1
高等院校药学类专业双语实验教材
ISBN 978-7-5214-0720-4

Ⅰ. ①药… Ⅱ. ①温… ②綦… Ⅲ. ①药物化学–化学实验–双语教学–高等学校–教材
Ⅳ. ①R914-33

中国版本图书馆 CIP 数据核字（2019）第 010248 号

美术编辑　陈君杞
版式设计　易维鑫

出版　**中国健康传媒集团** | 中国医药科技出版社
地址　北京市海淀区文慧园北路甲 22 号
邮编　100082
电话　发行：010-62227427　邮购：010-62236938
网址　www.cmstp.com
规格　787×1092mm ¹⁄₁₆
印张　5 ½
字数　116 千字
版次　2019 年 1 月第 1 版
印次　2019 年 1 月第 1 次印刷
印刷　三河市双峰印刷装订有限公司
经销　全国各地新华书店
书号　ISBN 978-7-5214-0720-4
定价　**16.00 元**

前　言

　　药物化学实验是药物化学课程的重要组成部分，其目的是通过实验加深理解药物化学的基本理论和基本知识，掌握药物合成的基本原理和基本方法，了解对药物进行结构修饰的基本方法，熟悉药品纯化精制的基本步骤和基本操作，进一步巩固有机化学实验的操作技术及有关理论知识，培养学生理论联系实际的作风、严谨求实的科学态度及创新能力。

　　本实验教材由三大部分组成，第一部分介绍了实验室的安全常识和基本知识；第二部分收集了 9 个药物合成实验，在实验内容上考虑到专业的差异性，我们选择了不同难度和实验时间长度不一的实验，可供不同专业、不同层次的学生选择使用；第三部分为附录，附有常用的实验技术和实验方法，供参考使用。

　　本教材具体分工如下：第一部分由綦慧敏编写；第二部分中，实验一和实验五由刘冬梅编写，实验二由贾海永编写，实验三由刘潇潇编写，实验四由孙延龙编写，实验六由曾现忠编写，实验七和第三部分由温新民编写，实验八由管华编写，实验九由闫玉刚编写，实验十由李伟编写，实验十一由王其宝编写。

　　为适应新世纪对新一代药学类专业人才的需求，本实验教材以综合实验为基础，突出创新和设计实验的重点。同时，本实验教材采用中英文对照编写，可以使学生的专业英语水平得以提高。在今后的使用过程中，我们仍要不断收集意见、总结经验，以便进一步提高完善。

编　者
2018 年 10 月

目　录

第一部分 药物化学实验基本知识

一、实验室安全及事故的预防与处理

药物化学是一门实践性很强的学科，因此，在进入实验室进行实验之前，要求参加实验者必须对实验课程的内容有充分的准备，要通晓实验室的一些基本规则，遵守实验室安全操作须知，避免可能发生的一些危险情况。

（一）眼睛安全防护

在实验室中，眼睛是最容易受到伤害的。飞溅出的腐蚀性化学药品和化学试剂，进入眼睛会引起灼伤和烧伤；在操作过程中，溅出的碎玻璃片或某些固体颗粒，也会使眼睛受到伤害；更有甚者，有可能发生的爆炸事故，更容易使眼睛受到损伤。因此在实验室中，最重要的是要佩戴合适的防护目镜。防护目镜一般是有机玻璃材质，并有护框，可以遮挡住整个眼睛。安全起见，在进入实验室后要养成戴防护目镜的习惯。

倘若有化学药品或酸、碱液溅入眼睛，应尽快用大量的水冲洗眼睛和脸部，并尽快到最近的医院进行治疗。若有固体颗粒或碎玻璃进入眼睛内，切记不要揉眼睛，立即去有关医院进行诊治。

（二）预防火灾

有机药物合成实验中，由于经常使用挥发性的、易燃性的各种有机试剂或溶剂，最容易发生的危险就是火灾。因此在实验中应严格遵守实验室的各项规章制度，以预防火灾的发生。

在实验室或实验大楼内禁止吸烟。实验室中使用明火时应考虑周围的环境，如周围有人使用易燃易爆溶剂时，应禁止明火。

一旦发生火灾，不要惊慌，须迅速切断电源、熄灭火源，并移开易燃物品，就近寻找灭火的器材，扑灭火苗。如容器中少量溶剂起火，可用石棉网、湿抹布或玻璃盖住容器口，扑灭火苗；其他着火，采用灭火器进行扑火，并立即报告有关部门或打 119 火警电话报警。

在实验中，万一衣服着火了，切勿奔跑，否则火借风势越烧越烈。可就近找到灭火喷淋器或自来水龙头，用水冲淋使火熄灭。

（三）伤、烫伤和试剂灼伤处理

1. 割伤 遇到割伤时，如无特定的要求，要用水充分清洗伤口，并取出伤口中碎玻璃或残留固体，用无菌的绷带或创可贴进行包扎、保护。大伤口应注意压紧伤口或血管，进行止血，并急送医疗部门进行处理。

2. 烫伤 因火焰或因触及灼热物体所致的小范围的轻度烫伤、烧伤，可通过立即将受伤部位浸入冷水或冰水中约 5 分钟以减轻疼痛。重度的大范围的烫伤或烧伤应立即去医疗部门进行救治。

3. 化学试剂 对于不同的化学试剂灼伤，处理方法不一样。

（1）酸 立即用大量水冲洗，再用 3%～5% 碳酸氢钠溶液淋洗 10～15 分钟。严重者将灼伤部位拭干包扎好，到医院治疗。

（2）碱 立即用大量水冲洗，再用 2% 醋酸溶液 25% 醋酸溶液或 1% 硼酸溶液淋洗，以中和碱，最后再水洗 10～15 分钟。

（3）溴 立即用大量水冲洗，再用 10% 硫代硫酸钠溶液淋洗或用湿的硫代硫酸钠纱布湿敷该灼伤处，至少 3 小时。

（4）有机物 用乙醇擦洗可以除去大部分有机物。然后再用肥皂和温水洗涤即可。

（四）中毒预防

有毒物质溅入口中尚未咽下者应立即吐出，用大量水冲洗口腔。如已吞下，应根据毒物性质进行解毒，并立即送有关医疗单位救治。

刺激性及神经性毒物中毒，先用牛奶或鸡蛋白使之冲淡或缓和，再设法催吐，使误入口中的毒物吐出，并送医院救治。

吸入气体中毒者，将中毒者移至室外通风处，解开衣领或纽扣，使其呼吸新鲜空气，必要时施行人工呼吸。

二、化学药品、试剂的储存及使用

（一）化学药品的储存

一般实验室中不应储存过多的化学药品和试剂，应实行需要多少，领用多少的原则。

在大多数情况下，实验室所用的化学药品都贮存在带磨口塞（最好是标准磨口）的玻璃瓶内，高黏度的液体放在广口瓶中，一般性液体存放在细颈瓶内，氢氧化钠和氢氧化钾溶液保存在带橡皮塞或塑料塞的瓶中。对于能够与玻璃发生反应的化合物（如氢氟酸），则使用塑料或金属容器，碱金属存放在煤油中，黄磷则需以水覆盖。

对光敏感的物质，包括醚在内，都有形成过氧化物的倾向，在光线的作用下更是如此，应将它们贮存在棕色玻璃瓶中。

对产生毒性或腐蚀性蒸气的物质（如溴、发烟硫酸、盐酸、氢氟酸）建议放在通风橱内专门的地方。

少量的或对潮湿气和空气敏感的物质常密封贮存于玻璃安瓿中。某些毒品（如氰化物、砷及其化合物等）应按有关部门的规定进行贮存。

（二）化学药品使用中注意的事项

有机溶剂具有易燃和有毒两个特点。

易燃的有机溶剂（特别是低沸点易燃溶剂）在室温时有较大的蒸气压，当空气中混杂易燃有机溶剂的蒸气达到某一极限时，遇到明火会立即发生燃烧爆炸。而且有机溶剂都较空气的密度大，会沿着桌面或地面飘移至较远处，或沉积在低洼处。因此，在实验室中用剩的火柴梗切勿乱丢，以免引起火灾。也不要将易燃溶剂倒入废物缸中，更不能用开口容器盛放易燃溶剂。

有机溶剂以较为隐蔽的方式产生对人的毒害，在使用中应注意最大限度地减少与有机溶剂的直接接触。不要掉以轻心。实验室中应充分通风。在正规、小心的操作下，有机溶剂不致造成任何健康问题。操作有毒试剂和物质时，必须戴橡皮手套或一次性塑料手套，操作后立即洗手。注意切勿让有毒物质触及五官或伤口。

三、废品的销毁

碎玻璃和其他锐角的废物不要丢入类似废纸篓的容器中，应该使用专门的废物箱。

不要把任何用剩的试剂倒回到试剂瓶中，因为这会对试剂造成污染，影响其他人的实验；更会由于操作疏忽导致错误引入异物，有时会发生剧烈的化学反应甚至会引起爆炸。

危险的废品，如会放出毒气或能够自燃的废品（活性镍、磷、碱金属等），决不能丢弃在废物箱或水槽中。不稳定的化学品和不溶于水或与水不混溶的溶液也禁止倒入下水道。应将它们分类集中后处理。对倒掉后能与水混溶，或能被水分解或腐蚀性液体，必须用大量的水冲洗。

金属钾或钠的残渣应分批小量地加到大量的乙醇中予以分解（操作时须戴防护目镜）。

四、实验的预习、记录和报告

在实验前，对所做的实验应该充分做好预习工作。预习工作包括反应的原理、可能发生的副反应、反应机制、实验操作的原理和方法、产物提纯的原理和方法、注意事项及实验中可能出现的危险及处置方法，应给出详细的报告。同时还要对化学试剂和溶剂的理化常数等要记录在案，以便查询。

做好实验记录和实验报告是每一个科研人员必备的基本素质。实验记录应记在专门的实验记录本上，实验记录本应有连续页码。所有观察到的现象、实验记录、原始数据、操作和后处理方法、步骤均应及时、准确，详细地记录在实验记录本上，并签名，以保证实验记录的完整性、连续性和原始性。将实验情况记录在便条纸、餐巾纸、纸巾等容易失落或损失的地方的任何做法都是错误的。

其中实验报告应按照规定的格式撰写，文前包括以下几个方面：实验题目、实验人、实验日期、室温等基本信息。正文包括以下几个方面：实验目的，实验原理，试剂或溶剂理化常数，试剂规格及用量，实验操作及实验现象，实验结果（包括产率、产品状态等）以及讨论部分。

第二部分　药物合成实验

实验一　阿司匹林（乙酰水杨酸）的合成

一、实验目的

1. 掌握酯化反应的原理及基本操作。
2. 巩固重结晶、熔点的测定、抽滤等操作。
3. 熟悉阿司匹林中杂质的来源及去除方法。

二、实验原理

阿司匹林（aspirin），又称乙酰水杨酸，为水杨酸类解热镇痛药。具有解热、镇痛、抗炎、抗风湿及抗血小板聚集等作用，临床常用于感冒发热、头痛、牙痛、神经痛、关节痛及类风湿关节炎等。近来发现阿司匹林能够抑制血小板中血栓素 A_2 的合成，抗血小板聚集，预防心血管疾病等。

阿司匹林为白色针状结晶或结晶性粉末，化学名为 2-乙酰氧基苯甲酸，熔点（mp.）135～140 ℃，分子式 $C_9H_8O_4$，分子量 180.16。易溶于乙醇，溶于三氯甲烷、乙醚、乙酸乙酯，微溶于水。阿司匹林的化学结构式为：

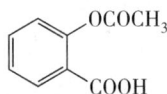

阿司匹林的合成通常以水杨酸为原料，经浓硫酸催化，与乙酸酐在酚羟基上发生酰化反应制备得到，其合成路线如下：

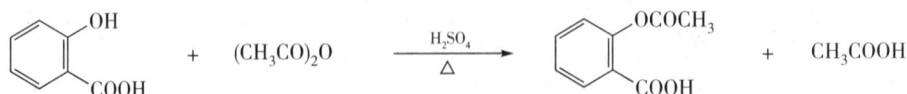

反应过程中，水杨酸分子之间可以发生缩合，生成少量聚合物。该聚合物不溶于碳酸氢钠溶液，而阿司匹林能与碳酸氢钠反应生成水溶性钠盐，可利用此性质把聚合物从阿司匹林中去除。

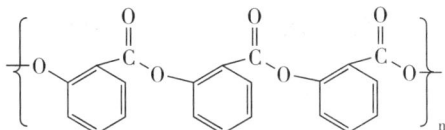

阿司匹林粗产品中还含有杂质水杨酸，该杂质可能由于乙酰化反应不完全或在分离步骤中发生水解而产生，可在各步纯化和产物的重结晶过程中除去。水杨酸含有酚羟基，可与 $FeCl_3$ 形成深色络合物，而乙酰水杨酸因酚羟基已被酰化，不与 $FeCl_3$ 显色，利用该方法可以检测阿司匹林粗品中的水杨酸。

三、仪器和试剂

仪器：磁力加热搅拌器，球形冷凝器，温度计，三颈瓶（250 ml），圆底烧瓶（100 ml），烧杯（250 ml），布氏漏斗，抽滤瓶。

试剂：水杨酸，乙酸酐，浓硫酸，饱和碳酸氢钠溶液，浓盐酸，乙酸乙酯，活性炭，乙醇，10% $FeCl_3$ 溶液。

四、实验步骤

（一）酯化

在装有球形冷凝器及温度计的 250 ml 三颈瓶中（注 1），依次加入水杨酸 10 g，乙酸酐 14 ml（注 2），浓硫酸 5～10 滴。磁力搅拌，油浴加热，维持反应温度为 70～75 ℃。反应 30 分钟，停止搅拌，将三颈瓶从油浴移出，室温冷却至 35～40 ℃后，将反应液倾入装有 200 ml 冷水的烧杯中，不断用玻璃棒搅拌，直至阿司匹林固体全部析出，抽滤，用少量冷水淋洗所得固体，压干，得阿司匹林粗品。

（二）精制

将所得阿司匹林粗品放入 150 ml 锥形瓶中，缓慢加入饱和碳酸氢钠水溶液 125 ml（注 3），搅拌到没有二氧化碳放出为止。抽滤，除去不溶物并用少量水洗涤。将所得滤液倒入 250 ml 烧杯中，冰浴冷却，向烧杯中滴加浓盐酸，同时用玻璃棒搅拌，调至 pH 为 2，溶液中有白色固体析出。抽滤，用冷水洗涤，尽量压干。

将所得固体置于附有球形冷凝器的 100 ml 圆底烧瓶中，加入少量乙酸乙酯，加热至阿司匹林全部溶解，稍冷，加入活性炭脱色 10 分钟，趁热抽滤，冷却至室温，析出白色结晶（注 4）。待结晶析出完全后，抽滤，干燥，得阿司匹林精品。称重，计算收率。

（三）结构确证

1. 标准物 TLC 对照法 取阿司匹林标准品及阿司匹林精品各 40 μg，分别置于点样板内，加入 2 滴无水乙醇溶解，点样于硅胶 GF254 高效预制薄层板上，以石油醚–乙酸乙酯–冰醋酸（12:6:0.1）为展开剂，紫外灯下观察，记录标准品与样品斑点位置，并计算 R_f 值。

2. 熔点的测定 取阿司匹林精品 5 mg，研成粉末，装于熔点管内，测定并记录阿司匹林的熔点。测定三次，取平均值。

（四）水杨酸杂质检测

取两只洁净试管，分别加入少量水杨酸和阿司匹林精品，各加入 1 ml 乙醇溶解后，分别加入一滴 10% $FeCl_3$ 溶液，盛水杨酸的试管中有红色或紫色出现，盛阿司匹林精品的试管中应为淡黄色或浅紫色。

五、注意事项

1. 乙酰化反应所用玻璃仪器均需干燥。

2. 乙酸酐有强烈乙酸味，易燃，有腐蚀性、催泪性，勿接触皮肤或眼睛，以防引起损伤。

3. 碳酸氢钠水溶液加到阿司匹林中，会产生大量的气泡，注意分批少量加入，边加边搅拌，防止气泡产生过多引起溶液外溢。

4. 如没有阿司匹林析出，可用玻璃棒轻轻摩擦锥形瓶的内壁，或加热将乙酸乙酯挥发一些，再冷却。

六、思考

1. 本实验乙酰化反应中所用仪器、量具为什么必须进行干燥？

2. 阿司匹林制备过程中加入少量浓硫酸的目的是什么？能否用其他酸代替？

3. 阿司匹林制备过程中可能发生哪些副反应？产生哪些副产物？

4. 阿司匹林精制过程中加入饱和碳酸氢钠的目的是什么？

5. 本实验中重结晶溶剂选择的依据是什么？通过该溶剂可以去除哪些杂质？

Experiment 1　Synthesis of Aspirin

1. Objective

1.1　To study the principle and the operation of esterifaction reaction.

1.2　To strenghthen the operations of recrystallization, melting point determination, and suction filtration.

1.3　To understand the source of the impurities in aspirin and learn how to remove them.

2. Principle

Aspirin, an antipyretic analgesic drug of salicylates, is also named as acetylsalicylic acid, which is used for the treatment of cold, headache, toothache, neuralgia, arthralgia and rheumatoid arthritis due to its beneficial effects of anti-pyretic analgesis, anti-inflammatory and anti-rheumatism. In recent years, it has been used for preventing cardiovascular events by virtue of its capacity of restraining the agglomeration of blood platelet by inhibiting the synthesis of TXA_2.

The aspirin is a white, needle-like crystal or crystalline powder with the chemical name of 2-acetoxybenzoic acid, melting point of $135\sim140$ ℃, formula of $C_9H_8O_4$ and molecular weight of 180.16. It is freely soluble in ethanol, soluble in chloroform, ether and ethyl acetate, and slightly soluble in water. The compound is represented by the following structural formula:

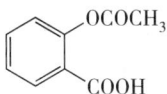

The synthesis of aspirin involves a simple condensation reaction between acetic anhydride and hydroxy group on salicylic acid in the presence of a catalytic amount of H_2SO_4. The synthetic route is as following:

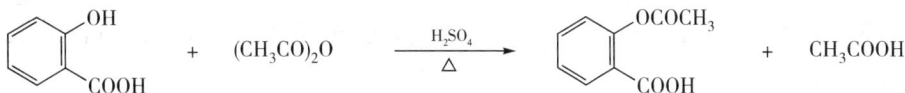

During the reaction, salicylic acid can condensate with itself to produce a polymer byproduct. Comparing with the polymer, the aspirin has a free carboxylic acid group. Therefore, the aspirin can react with $NaHCO_3$ and form a water-soluble sodium salt. However, the polymer can not react with $NaHCO_3$, which makes it possible to separate the polymer from aspirin.

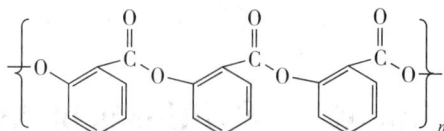

Another impurity in the aspirin is salicylic acid which may be from the unreacted material or the hydrolysis product of aspirin. It can be removed in the process of purification and recrystallization. The hydroxy group on salicylic acid can react with ferric chloride and form deep colour complex. However, the reaction can not arise because the hydroxy group in aspirin has been acelated and is not free.

3. Apparatus and Materials

Apparatus：magnetic heating stirrer, condenser-Allihn type, thermometer, three necked flask (250 ml), round bottom flask (100 ml), beaker (250 ml), Busher funnel, suction flask.

Materials：salicylic acid, acetic anhydride, concentrated sulfuric acid, saturated sodium bicarbonate aqueous solution, concentrated hydrochloric acid, ethyl acetate, active carbon.

4. Procedures

4.1　The esterification of salicylic acid

10 g of salicylic acid, 14 ml of acetic anhydride and 5～10 drops of concentrated sulfuric acid are added into a 250 ml three necked flask equipped with a reflux condenser and thermometer (Note 5.1 and 5.2). The reaction mixture is heated on an oil bath to 70～75 ℃ under magnetic stirring. 30 min later, the stirrer is stopped. The reaction mixture is moved out the bath, cooled to about 35～40 ℃, then poured into 200 ml of cold water in a beaker. Aspirin is precipitated little by little under constantly stirring with a glass rod. After being filtrated and washed with cold water, the crude aspirin is obtained.

4.2　The purification of crude aspirin

The crude aspirin is put into a 150 ml beaker, and 125 ml of saturated sodium bicarbonate aqueous solution is added. Keep stirring until without release of carbon dioxide. Filter off the solids and wash with a small amount of water. The filtrate solution is poured into a 250 ml beaker and added concentrated hydrochloric acid until the pH value gets to 2 (Note 5.3). The resultant white solid is washed with cold water and filtered under reduced pressure.

The above product is put into a 100 ml round bottom flask equipped with a spherical condenser, and small quantities of ethyl acetate is added to dissolve the solid under heating condition. After cooling down the solution to about 70～80 ℃, active carbon is added and kept boiling for 10 min, then immediately filtered. The white crystal will generate completely when the solution is cooled to room temperature (Note 5.4). Purified aspirin is obtained after the crystal is filtered and dried. Finally, the theoretical yield is calculated.

4.3　The identification of aspirin

4.3.1　Thin Layer chromatography (TLC)　Place 40 μg of standard aspirin and your purified aspirin separately in the spot plate and dissolve in two drops of ethanol. With a separate spotter for each compound, load the samples on a TLC plate. The eluting solution is a 12:6:0.1 mixture of petroleum ether, ethyl acetate and acetic acid. Visualize the eluted compounds on the plate using UV light, circle any spots observed with your pencil and note the colors and intensities of each spot. Measure the distance from the origin to the center of each spot and also the distance from the origin to the top of the solvent front. Use these values to calculate the R_f values for each spot.

4.3.2　Melting point analysis　Place 5 mg of your purified aspirin into the well of a spot plate. Use the bottom of a test tube to grind into a fine powder. Prepare a sample for melting point analysis by inserting a small amount of your crystals into closed end capillary tubes and place this in the melting point apparatus. Record your melting range of each sample. Values are the means of three replicates.

4.4　The determination of salicylic acid

Place a spatula tip of salicylic acid and purified aspirin in two clean test tubes and add 1 ml of ethanol. After the solid has been dissolved completely, add a drop of ferric chloride (10%). The tube containing salicylic acid will turn red or purple color. The other tube containing purified aspirin will remain yellow or turn light purple color. If it is the latter one, it indicates salicylic acid remains in your recrystallization.

5. Notes

5.1　All glasswares used in acelate reaction must be dried.

5.2　Acetic anhydride is an irritant and combustible liquid with a very pungent, penetrating, vinegar-like odor. Don't contact your eyes and skin for fear of hurt.

5.3　Plenty of bubbles will be generated during the process of mixing saturated sodium bicarbonate with aspirin. Add in several batches and stir continuously to avoid overflowing.

5.4　If no aspirin solid appears, we may scrape inside the flask gently with a glass rod or evaporate some ethyl acetate to form the crystal.

6. Questions

6.1　Why must you dry the glasswares used in the acelate reaction?

6.2　What is the purpose of adding concentrated sulfuric acid into the reaction mixture? Could it be substituted by other acids?

6.3　What side reactions will occur in the reaction? What are the byproducts?

6.4   What is the purpose of adding saturated sodium bicarbonate during the purification process of aspirin?

6.5   What is the principles for the recrystallization solvent in the experiment? What imputities can be removed by the solvent?

实验二　盐酸普鲁卡因的合成

一、实验目的

1. 根据水与二甲苯共沸的原理，掌握分水器的使用和酯化脱水反应的操作。
2. 通过局部麻醉药盐酸普鲁卡因的合成，掌握铁粉还原反应的操作。
3. 通过对盐酸普鲁卡因的精制，掌握盐析等分离方法的操作。

二、实验原理

盐酸普鲁卡因为局部麻醉药，作用强，毒性低。临床上主要用于浸润、脊椎和传导麻醉。盐酸普鲁卡因的化合物名为对氨基苯甲酸2－二乙胺基乙酯盐酸盐，化学结构为：

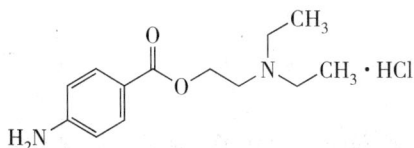

本品为白色细微针状结晶或结晶性粉末，无臭，味微苦而麻。熔点为153～157 ℃。易溶于水，溶于乙醇，微溶于三氯甲烷，几乎不溶于乙醚。

本品以对硝基苯甲酸为原料，经过酯化及还原反应得到盐酸普鲁卡因粗品，再经过盐析等分离方法进行精制。

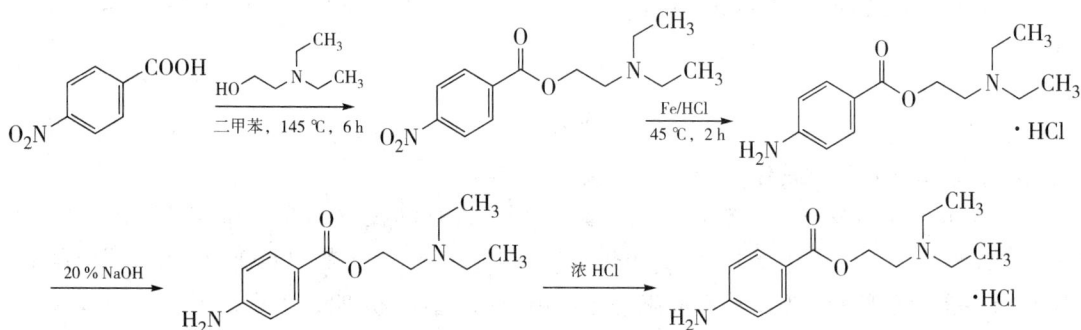

三、仪器和试剂

仪器：磁力加热搅拌器，球形冷凝器，温度计，三颈瓶（250 ml），圆底烧瓶（100 ml），烧杯（250 ml），布氏漏斗，抽滤瓶。

试剂：对硝基苯甲酸，β－二乙胺基乙醇，二甲苯，3% HCl，20% NaOH，活化铁粉，10% Na_2S，活性炭，浓 HCl，乙醇，连二亚硫酸钠（保险粉）。

四、实验步骤

（一）对硝基苯甲酸二乙胺基乙醇酯（俗称硝基卡因）的制备

取 500 ml 三颈或双颈瓶，装入温度计、回流冷凝分水器和搅拌子，将对硝基苯甲酸（30 g，0.18 mol）溶于 190 ml 二甲苯中（注1），在搅拌下加入 β-二乙胺基乙醇（22 g，0.188 mol），加热回流反应 6 小时（维持瓶内 145 ℃，油浴温度约为 180 ℃）（注2），反应完毕，冷却至室温析出固体（注3）。将上清液用倾泻法转移到减压蒸馏瓶中，用水泵减压蒸馏除去二甲苯，将剩余残液与反应瓶中的固体合并，加入 3% HCl 210 ml 溶解，滤除未反应的对硝基苯甲酸，滤液用 20% NaOH 调至 pH 4～4.2，进行下一步还原反应。

注意事项

1. 羧酸与醇的酯化反应为可逆反应，通过水与二甲苯共沸以及水密度大的原理，利用分水器将反应瓶中生成的水移去，使酯化反应趋于完全。酯化反应中所用的仪器和原料须提前干燥。

2. 由于教学需要，将反应时间缩短为 6 小时（生产反应时间为 19 小时），如果延长反应时间，收率可能提高。

3. 如果反应完毕后不冷却，直接减压蒸除二甲苯，析出的固体较多，易爆沸。

（二）普鲁卡因的制备

取 500 ml 三颈瓶，装入温度计和搅拌子，加入上一步制备的硝基卡因盐酸盐溶液，在室温搅拌下缓慢分批加入活化铁粉（注1），反应温度自动上升（注2），加毕，保持 45 ℃ 继续反应 2 小时。抽滤，少量水洗涤滤渣两次；首先用稀 HCl 调节滤液 pH 值为 5，再用 10% Na_2S 调 pH 至 7.8～8。再次抽滤，用少量水洗涤滤渣两次，并用稀 HCl 调节滤液至 pH=6。加入少量活性炭，于 50～60 ℃ 搅拌 10 分钟（注3），再次抽滤，用少量水洗涤滤渣一次，将滤液冷却至 10 ℃ 以下，并用 20% NaOH 调至 pH 9.5～10.5，析出固体，抽滤并压干备用。

注意事项

1. 为了除去铁粉表面的铁锈，首先进行活化：将 1 ml 浓盐酸溶于 150 ml 水中，加入 70 g 铁粉后煮沸；用水洗铁粉至中性，置水中待用。

2. 此反应为放热反应，铁粉必须少量分批加入，避免剧烈反应。温度控制在 45 ℃ 为宜，并注意反应液颜色变化 [绿($Fe(OH)_2$)→棕($Fe(OH)_3$)→黑(Fe_3O_4)]。若一段时间后，反应仍不能成棕黑色，表示反应尚未完全，可补加适量铁粉继续反应。

3. Na_2S 除去多余的铁粉，且过量的 Na_2S 被酸化后可形成胶体硫，并被活性炭吸附。

（三）盐酸普鲁卡因制备

1. 成盐 将上步制备的普鲁卡因置于干燥的小烧杯中（注1），在冰浴下缓慢滴加浓 HCl 调至 pH 5.5（注2），加热至 60 ℃ 后加入精制的氯化钠至饱和（注3），继续升温至 60 ℃ 后加入适量保险粉（注4），于 65～70 ℃ 趁热抽滤，冷却滤液至 10 ℃ 以下，抽滤，得盐酸普鲁卡因粗品。

2. 精制 将上步制备的粗品置于干燥的小烧杯中，滴加蒸馏水，并在 70 ℃ 时恰好溶解为止，加入适量的保险粉，并于 70 ℃继续反应 10 分钟。趁热过滤，将滤液冰浴下冷却，使结晶析出完全。过滤，用少量冷乙醇洗涤两次，干燥，称重，计算总收率。测定熔点：153～157 ℃。

注意事项

1. 盐酸普鲁卡因易溶于水，所用仪器须干燥，否则影响收率。

2. 严格控制 pH，防止芳胺基成盐。

3. 利用盐析法，加入精制氯化钠使之从水中分离。

4. 保险粉为强还原剂，可除去有色杂质，并防止芳胺基被氧化，但过量会导致成品含硫量不合格，用量应控制在 1% 以下。

五、思考

1. 在盐酸普鲁卡因的制备中，为何先酯化再还原，能否反之，为什么？

2. 酯化反应有什么特点，在反应中如何控制，二甲苯在本实验中的作用是什么，脱水剂应该具备哪些条件？

3. 试说明铁粉还原的反应历程，以及采用铁粉还原硝基化合物在电解质存在下的主要影响因素有哪些？

4. 还原反应结束后加入硫化钠的目的是什么？

Experiment 2　Synthesis of Procaine Hydrochloride

1. Objective

1.1　According to the azeotropic principle of water and xylene, master the use of water separator and the operation of esterification dehydration reaction.

1.2　Mastery learning reduction reaction by iron powder through the synthesis of local anesthetics procaine hydrochloride.

1.3　Mastering the operation of salting-out separation method through the refining of procaine hydrochloride.

2. Principle

Procaine hydrochloride, a local anesthetic, has a strong effect with low toxicity. It is mostly used to local anaesthesia of soak, acantha andconduction. The chemical name of procaine hydrochloride is 2-(diethylamino) ethyl 4-aminobenzoate hydrochloride, and the structure of which is as follow:

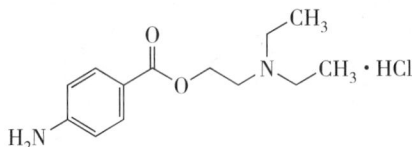

This product is a white fine needle crystals or crystal powder, odourless, and has a bitter and numbing taste. The melting point of this product is $153\sim157\ ℃$. It could easily dissolve into water, and which is soluble in ethanol, less soluble in chloroform, but hardly dissolve in diethyl ether.Raw procaine hydrochloride was prepared from p-nitrobenzoic acid through esterification and reduction reaction, and was further refined by salting-out separation methods.

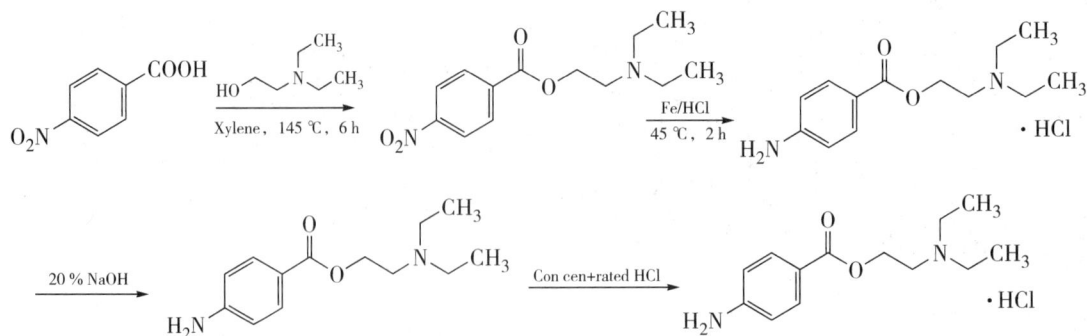

3. Apparatus and Materials

Apparatus: magnetic heating stirrer, condenser-allihn type, thermometer, three necked flask (250 ml), round bottom flask (100 ml), beaker (250 ml), Busher funnel, suction flask.

Materials: *p*-nitrobenzoic acid, *β*-(diethylamino) ethanol, concentrated hydrochloric acid, xylene , 3% HCl , active ferrous , 20% NaOH , active carbon, ethanol, sodium dithionite.

4. Procedures

4.1   Preparation of *p*-nitrobenzoic acid-*β*-(diethylamino) ethyl ester

p-nitrobenzoic acid (30 g), β−(diethylamino) ethanol (22 g) and xylene (190 ml) were added to a 500 ml three necked flask equipped with thermometer, water segregator, condenser and a stir bar (Note a). The reaction mixture was refluxed in an oil bath (the outside temperature is 180 ℃, but 145 ℃ inside) for 6 hours (Note b). After reaction, the reaction mixture was cooled to room temperature and solid was precipitated (Note c). Then the reaction solvent was poured into a distilled flask, and the xylene was evaporated under reduced-pressure by water pump. The residue was combined with the solid in the reaction flask, and was dissolved by 210 ml 3% HCl, which was filtered to remove the unreacted *p*-nitrobenzoic acid. The filtrate was further adjusted pH value to 4~4.2 with 20% NaOH, which was saved for the next step of reduction reaction.

Notes

a. The esterification reaction of carboxylic acid and alcohol is a reversible reaction. As the density water is larger than xylene, water separator is used to remove the produced water continuously to prompt the reaction mostly completed according to the azeotropic principle of water and xylene. Therefore, the reagents and apparatus used in the experiment need to be dried beforehand.

b. Considering the need in teaching experiment, the reaction time is reduced to 6 hours (19 hours are needed in the production). If the reaction time is prolonged, the yield will increase.

c. It is not allowed to evaporate the xylene directly without cooling, as too much solid will block the capillary, which resulted in inconvenience.

4.2   Synthesis of *p*-aminobenzoic acid 2-(diethylamino) ethyl ester

The filtrate prepared above was added to a 500 ml three necked flask with stirrer and thermometer. Then the active ferrous (Note a) was slowly added in batches under temperature with stirring, meanwhile the temperature of the reactant would raised automatically (Note b). Please control the reaction temperature about 45 ℃ and react for 2 hours after completely added. Upon completion of the reaction, the mixture solution was filtrated, then the residue was washed twice with little water, and the filtrate was adjusted pH to 5 with diluted hydrochloride acid. After that the saturated sodium sulfide solvent was added dropwise to adjust the pH to 7.8~8.0. The mixture was filtrated again, the residue was asol washed twice with a little amount of water again, and the filtrate was acidified to pH 6 with diluted hydrochloride acid. Some active carbon was added and reacted under 50~60 ℃ for 10 min (Note c). Then the mixture solution was filtrated, and the residue was washed with little water. At last, the filtrate was cooled below 10 ℃ and basified with sodium hydroxyl to pH 9.5~10.5, and the solid precipitation was filtrated and obtained.

Notes:

a. In order to remove the rust on the ferrous powder surface, the ferrous powder was activated first. Methods: ferrous powder (70 g), water (100 ml) and concentrated hydrochloride acid (0.7 ml) were heated together to a bit boiling state, which were washed with water to neutral and deposited in the water on standby.

b. As it is an exothermic reaction, the ferrous powder should be slowly added in batches to prevent a blast reaction. It is better to control the reaction temperature about 45 ℃. During the reaction, the colour of reaction mixture changed from green ($Fe(OH)_2$) to brown ($Fe(OH)_3$) and black (Fe_3O_4) finally. If the brownish black color did not occur, the reaction might not have completed, and additional ferrous powder should be added to continue the reaction.

c. Excess ferrous powder was removed by Na_2S. And excess of Na_2S would form sulphur after acidification, which would be absorbed by the active carbon.

4.3　Synthesis of procaine hydrochloride

4.3.1　Salification　The solid of procaine prepared above was added to a small dry beaker (Note 1), and concentrated acid was added dropwise to adjust the pH to 5.5 slowly under ice-bath (Note 2). After it was heated to 60 ℃, refined sodium chloride was added to make saturated solution (Note 3). Some sodium dithionite was added when the mixture was heated to 60 ℃ again (Note 4). The mixture was filtered under 65~70 ℃, and the filtrate was cooled to 10 ℃ below. Filtered and the crude of procaine hydrochloride was obtained.

4.3.2　Refinement　The crude of procaine hydrochloride prepared above was added to a small dry beaker, distilled water was added dropwise to just dissolve the solid at 70 ℃. Appropriate amount of sodium dithionite was added and reacted for 10 min under 70 ℃. After hot filtration, the filtrate was cooled under ice-bath to complete the crystallization. Filtering, and the solid was washed twice time with little cold ethanol. Drying, weighing, and calculating total yield.Determination of melting point: 153~157 ℃.

Notes:

a. As procaine hydrochlorid is well solubility in water, all the apparatus must be dried. Otherwise, it will affect the yield.

b. Strictly control the pH to prevent the salts formation of the aromatic amino.

c. The refined sodium chloride was added to separated procaine hydrochlorid from water using the method of salting-out.

d. The sodium dithionite was a strong reductant, which could prevent the oxidation of aromatic amino group and remove the colored by-product from white product at the same time. However, excess amount of sodium dithionite would result in disqualification, so the dosage of which should be controlled below 1%.

5. Questions

5.1　Why esterification of the *p*-nitrobenzoic acid is prior to the reduction reaction in the preparation of procaine hydrochloride. Could the sequence be reverse?

5.2　Why xylene was added as solvent in the esterification?What is the distinguishing feature of esterification reaction, and how to control it in the reaction. What is the role of xylene in this experiment, and what conditions dehydrant should have?

5.3　What is the reaction mechanism of iron powder reduction. What is the main influencing factors of the reduction reaction of iron powder with nitro compounds in the presence of electrolytes?

5.4　Why the sodium sulfide was added after reduction reaction?

实验三 贝诺酯的合成

一、实验目的

1. 通过乙酰水杨酰氯的制备，掌握氯化反应的一般方法及基本操作。
2. 通过贝诺酯的合成，了解拼合原理在药物化学结构修饰中的应用。

二、实验原理

贝诺酯为一种新型非甾体解热镇痛抗炎药，由阿司匹林和对乙酰氨基酚经拼合原理制成，既能保留原药的解热镇痛功能，又能减小原药的毒副作用，并能发挥协同作用。适用于急、慢性风湿性关节炎，风湿痛，感冒发烧，头痛及神经痛等。贝诺酯的化学名为 2 - 乙酰氧基苯甲酸 - 乙酰胺基苯酯，化学结构式为：

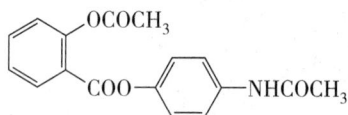

合成路线如下：

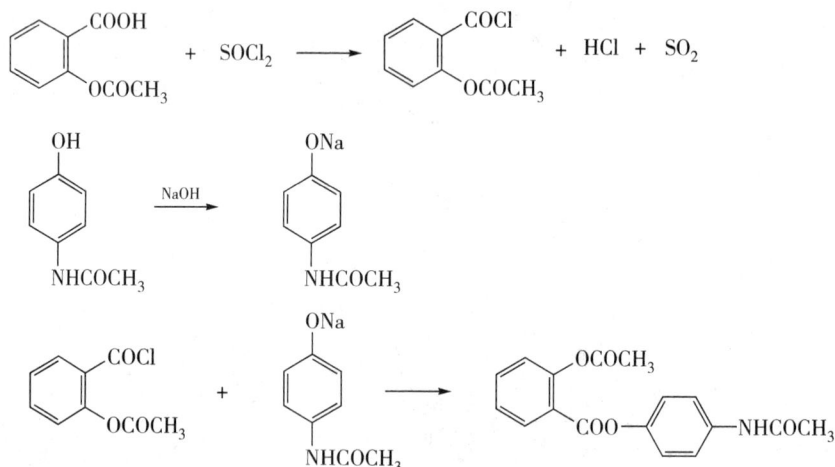

三、仪器和试剂

仪器：磁力加热搅拌器，球形冷凝器，温度计，三颈瓶（250 ml），圆底烧瓶（100 ml），烧杯（250 ml），布氏漏斗，抽滤瓶，氯化钙干燥管。

试剂：吡啶，阿司匹林，氯化亚砜，无水丙酮，扑热息痛，氢氧化钠，活性炭，乙醇。

四、实验步骤

（一）乙酰水杨酰氯的制备

在干燥的 100 ml 圆底烧瓶中，依次加入吡啶 2 滴，阿司匹林 10 g，氯化亚砜 5.5 ml，立即安装球形冷凝器（冷凝器顶端附有氯化钙干燥管，干燥管连有导气管，导气管另一端通入水池下水口）。将圆底烧瓶置于油浴上缓慢加热至 70 ℃（10～15 分钟），并维持油浴温度在 70 ℃±2 ℃，反应 70 min，冷却，加入无水丙酮 10 ml，将反应液转移到干燥的 100 ml 滴液漏斗中，混合均匀，密闭备用。

（二）贝诺酯的制备

在装有磁子及温度计的 250 ml 三颈瓶中，加入对乙酰氨基酚 10 g、水 50 ml。将三颈瓶置于冰水浴中冷却至 10 ℃左右，在搅拌下滴加氢氧化钠溶液（氢氧化钠 3.6 g 溶解于 20 ml 水配成）。滴加完毕，控制温度在 8～12 ℃，剧烈搅拌下缓慢滴加上步实验制得的乙酰水杨酰氯丙酮溶液（约 20 分钟滴完）。滴加完毕，调至 pH≥10，控制温度在 8～12 ℃，继续搅拌反应 60 分钟。抽滤，水洗至中性，得粗品。

（三）精制

在装有球形冷凝器的 100 ml 圆底瓶中，加入 5 g 粗品，10 倍量（w/v）95%乙醇，在水浴上加热溶解。稍冷，加适量活性炭脱色（活性炭用量根据粗品颜色而定），加热回流 30 分钟，趁热抽滤（布氏漏斗、抽滤瓶应预热）。将滤液趁热转移至烧杯中，自然冷却，待结晶完全析出后，抽滤，压干；用少量乙醇洗涤两次（母液回收），压干，干燥，计算收率，mp.175～178 ℃。

五、注意事项

1. 二氯亚砜是由羧酸制备酰氯最常用的氯化试剂，价格便宜且沸点低，生成的副产物均为挥发性气体，所得酰氯产品易于纯化。二氯亚砜遇水可分解为二氧化硫和氯化氢，因此所用仪器均需干燥；加热时不能用水浴。阿司匹林需在 60 ℃干燥 4 小时。

2. 吡啶作为催化剂，用量不宜过多，否则影响产品的质量。

3. 制得的酰氯不应久置。

4. 严格控制反应温度：酰氯化反应时，温度不能超过 80 ℃；缩合酯化时，温度控制在 10 ℃左右。

六、思考

1. 制备乙酰水杨酰氯的操作上应注意哪些事项？

2. 制备贝诺酯时，为什么先制备对乙酰氨基酚钠，再与乙酰水杨酰氯进行酯化，而不直接酯化？

Experiment 3　Synthesis of Benorilate

1. Objective

1.1　To grasp the basic principle and general procedure of chlorination through the synthesis of acetylsalicyloyl chloride.

1.2　To grasp the combination principles and their application in chemical structure modification through the synthesis of benorilate.

2. Principle

Benorilate is a nonsteroidalantipyretic, analgesic and anti-inflammatory drug, which is an ester-linked codrug of aspirin with paracetamol.Compared to the original drug, benorilate retains the antipyretic and analgesic function, reduces the side effects, and also plays synergy activity. Benorilate is used in the treatment of the acute and chronic rheumatoid arthritis, rheumatism, cold fever, headache and neuralgia.The chemical name of benorilate is 2-acetoxy benzoic acid-acetamido phenyl ester, and the chemical structure is shown as below:

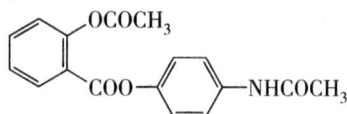

The synthetic route is shown as below:

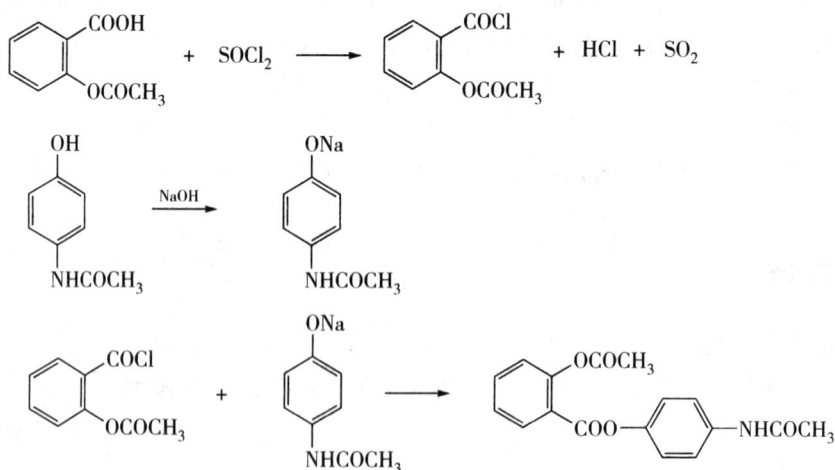

3. Apparatus and Materials

Apparatus: magnetic heating stirrer, condenser-Allihn type, thermometer, three necked flask（250 ml）, round bottom flask（100 ml）, beaker（250 ml）, Busher funnel, suction flask, calcium chloride drying tube.

Materials：pyridine, aspirin , thionyl chloridewere , anhydrous acetone, paracetamol, sodium hydroxide , active carbon, ethanol.

4. Procedures

4.1　Synthesis of acetylsalicyloyl chloride

In a dried 100 ml round-bottom flask, 2 drops of pyridine, 10 g of aspirin and 5.5 ml of thionyl chloridewere added successively, and quickly joined a spherical condenser (top equipped with calcium chloride drying tube which is connected to an airway, whose other end linking into the pool sewer). The mixture was slowly heat (10~15 min) to 70 ℃ in the oil bath.Keep the temperature at 70 ℃±2 ℃ for 70 min.Cool down.Add 10 ml of anhydrous acetone into the reaction solution, then pour the mixture into a dried 100 ml dropping funnel, mix well, standby.

4.2　The preparation of Benorilate

In a 250 ml three-necked round-bottom flask equipped with stirrer and thermometer, 10 g of paracetamol and 50 ml of water were added. Cool down the mixture to 10 ℃ in the ice water bath,thenadded 20ml sodium hydroxide solution (containing 3.6 g of sodium hydroxide) dropwisely into the mixture. After that dropwisely added the acetylsalicyloyl chloride acetone solution (prepared in step 4.1) under vigorous stirring at 8~12 ℃(in 20 min). The pH of the solution was adjusted to ≥10. Continue to react for 60 minutes at 8~12 ℃. The reaction solution was filtrated, washed with water, and the crude product was obtained.

4.3　Refinement

In a 100 ml round-bottom flask equipped with spherical condenser, 5 g of crude product and 10 volume folds (*w/v*) 95% ethanol were added respectively, then heated in the water bath until the crude product dissolved. Cool down. Add activated carbon, and reflux for 30 min. Filtrate while the reaction solution was hot.Transfer the filtration into a beaker, and cooled. After crystallization precipitated completely, filtrate. The crystallization was pressed, washed twice with a small amount of ethanol, and dried.Calculate the yield, and measure the melting point (mp. 153~157 ℃).

5. Notes

5.1　Thionyl chloride is one of the most common chlorination reagents used in the preparation of acyl chloride.It is cheap and has low boiling point.The resulting acyl chloride production is easy to purify because the by-products are volatile gases. In the presence of water, thionyl chloride can be decomposed into sulfur dioxide and hydrogen chloride, so the instruments used must be dried and be heated in oil bath, rather than in water bath. Aspirin should be dried at 60 ℃ for 4 h.

5.2　The amount of pyridine as a catalyst should not be too much, otherwise it will affect the quality of the product.

5.3   The product acyl chloride should not be set for a long time.

5.4   Strict control the reaction temperature: in acyl chloride reaction,the temperature can not exceed 80 ℃; in condensation esterification, the temperature should be at 10 ℃.

6. Questions

6.1   What are the precautionsduring the preparation of acetylsalicyloyl chloride?

6.2   In benorilate preparation, acetylaminophen is prepared as acetylaminophensodium before esterification with acetylsalicyloyl chloride, rather than direct esterification, why?

实验四 苯佐卡因的合成

一、实验目的

1. 掌握苯佐卡因合成的基本过程。
2. 掌握氧化、酯化及还原反应的原理及操作方法。
3. 掌握蒸馏、抽滤、回流、洗涤、干燥、熔点测定等基本操作。

二、实验原理

苯佐卡因（benzocaine）是对氨基苯甲酸乙酯的通用名称，可作为局部麻醉药。外用为撒布剂，用于手术后创伤止痛、溃疡痛、一般性瘙痒等。苯佐卡因化学名为对氨基苯甲酸乙酯，化学结构式为：

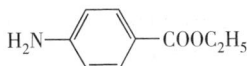

$$H_2N-\!\!\!\bigcirc\!\!\!-COOC_2H_5$$

苯佐卡因为白色结晶性粉末，味微苦而麻；mp. 88～90 ℃；易溶于乙醇，极微溶于水。合成路线如下：

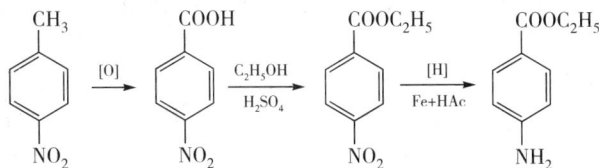

三、仪器和试剂

仪器：磁力加热搅拌器，球形冷凝器，温度计，三颈瓶（250 ml），圆底烧瓶（100 ml），烧杯（250 ml），布氏漏斗，抽滤瓶。

试剂：对硝基甲苯，重铬酸钠，浓硫酸，15%硫酸，5%氢氧化钠溶液，无水乙醇，碳酸钠，95%乙醇，冰醋酸，铁粉，活性炭，50%乙醇。

四、实验步骤

（一）对硝基苯甲酸的制备（氧化）

本实验采用机械搅拌装置，在装有温度计和球型冷凝器的 250 ml 三颈瓶中加入 8 g 研碎的对硝基甲苯、23.6 g 重铬酸钠和 50 ml 水，开动搅拌；用滴液漏斗滴加 32 ml 浓硫酸，随着浓硫酸的加入氧化反应随之开始。反应温度迅速上升，药液颜色逐渐变深，注意要严格控制滴加浓硫酸的速度。严防反应混合物温度高于回流温度，滴加时间约 20 到 30 分钟。滴加完毕，打开油浴锅加热，保持反应液微沸 60～90 分钟。停止加热冷却后慢慢加入 80 ml

冷水，然后关闭搅拌器，将混合物抽滤，残渣用 45 ml 水洗涤 3 次。粗制的对硝基苯甲酸为深黄色固体。将固体放入 100 ml 烧杯中，向烧杯中加入 76 ml 5%氢氧化钠溶液，温热不超过 60 ℃，使粗产物溶解，冷却后抽滤。在玻璃棒搅拌下，将滤液慢慢倒入盛有 60 ml 15%硫酸的另一个烧杯中，浅黄色沉淀立即析出。用试纸检验溶液是否呈酸性，呈酸性后抽滤，固体用少量水洗涤，抽滤，干燥得本品，计算收率。

（二）对硝基苯甲酸乙酯的制备（酯化）

在干燥的 250 ml 圆底烧瓶中放置对硝基苯甲酸 6 g、20 ml 无水乙醇，逐渐滴加入浓硫酸 2 ml，混匀后投入沸石，装上附有氯化钙干燥管的球型冷凝器，水浴加热回流 1～1.5 小时，将反应液趁热倒入装有 85 ml 冷水的 250 ml 烧杯中，搅动，加入碳酸钠固体粉末，至液面有少许白色沉淀出现时慢慢加入 5%碳酸钠溶液 10 ml，使溶液对 pH 试纸呈中性，抽滤，滤渣用水洗至中性，干燥，计算收率。

（三）对氨基苯甲酸乙酯的制备（还原）

在装有温度计及球型冷凝器的 100 ml 三颈瓶中，加入对硝基苯甲酸乙酯 6 g 和 95%乙醇 35 ml、2.5 ml 冰醋酸和铁粉 8.6 g，激烈搅拌下加热至 95～98 ℃，回流反应 90 分钟。稍冷，在搅拌下，分次加入温热的碳酸钠饱和溶液（由碳酸钠 3 g 和水 30 ml 配成），搅拌片刻，立即抽滤，滤液冷却后析出结晶，抽滤，产品用稀乙醇洗涤，干燥得粗品。

（四）精制

将苯佐卡因粗品置于 100 ml 圆底瓶中，加入 50%乙醇，在水浴上加热至其溶解。稍冷，加活性炭脱色，加热回流 20 分钟，趁热抽滤。将滤液趁热转移至烧杯中，冷却，待结晶完全析出后，抽滤，用 50%乙醇洗涤 2 次，抽滤，干燥，测熔点，计算收率。

（五）结构确证

1. 标准物 TLC 对照法。
2. 红外吸收光谱法。
3. 核磁共振光谱法。

五、注意事项

1. 本氧化反应十分激烈。采用机械搅拌和滴加硫酸的方法可使反应较平稳、安全。装置安装完毕后应经教师检查无误后再加料使用。

2. 滴液漏斗在使用前要检查其密封性是否完好。

3. 若滴加硫酸时烧瓶内有较多白色烟雾或火花出现，则应迅速减慢或暂停滴加，必要时用冷水浴冷却烧瓶。

4. 加浓硫酸时要慢，且不断振荡烧瓶使之在反应液中分散均匀，以防加热后引起碳化。

5. 必须剧烈振摇，使油层乳化，这样冷却后析出的结晶颗粒细，以后用碳酸钠处理易除去酸；否则会结成硬块，用碳酸钠不易处理。

6. 对硝基苯甲酸加入时反应放热，如加料速度快，则易致冲料。

7. 铁粉重，必须剧烈搅拌，才能使之不至于沉积在瓶底，使反应完全。

8. 为使产品少受损失，可采用分步抽滤的方法。即在有产品析出后，先滤集之，再将滤液加酸，如此反复抽滤，至无沉淀析出为止。

六、思考

1. 为什么酯化反应需要无水操作？
2. 还原反应的原理是什么？

Experiment 4　Synthesis of Benzocaine

1. Objective

1.1　To study the basic process of the synthesis of benzocaine.

1.2　To study the principle of oxidation, esterification and reduction reaction and operation methods.

1.3　To study the distillation, reflux, filtration, washing and drying, melting point and other basic operations.

2. Principle

Benzocaine is a common name for parathesin which could be used as a local anesthetic. It was used for postoperative trauma, pain relief, sore pain, general itching and so on. The chemical name of benzocaine is ethyl-4-aminobenzoate, and chemical structure is as follow:

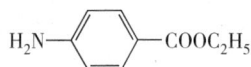

$$H_2N-\!\!\!\!\diagup\!\!\!\!\diagdown\!\!\!\!-COOC_2H_5$$

Benzocaine is white crystal powder and has a mildly bitter flavor.Its melting point is between 88~90 ℃, and it is soluble in ethanol but very slightly soluble in water. The synthetic route is as follow:

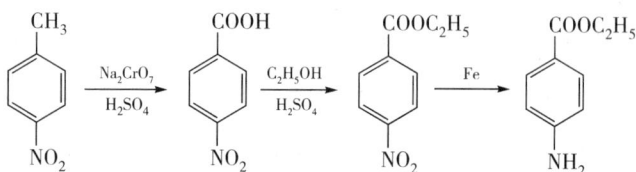

3. Apparatus and Materials

Apparatus: magnetic heating stirrer, condenser-Allihn type, thermometer, three necked flask (250 ml), round bottom flask (100 ml), beaker (250 ml), Busher funnel, suction flask.

Materials: p-nitrotoluene, sodium dichromate, concentrated sulfuric acid, odium hydroxide solution (5%), 15% H_2SO_4, absolute ethanol, sodium carbonate, ethanol (95%), acetic acid, iron powder, active carbon.

4. Procedures

4.1　Synthesis of p-nitrobenzoic acid (Oxidation)

8 g p-nitrotoluene, 23.6 g sodium dichromate ($Na_2CrO_7 \cdot 2H_2O$) and 50 ml water were

added to a 250 ml three necked flask equipped with mechanical stirrer and condenser. 32 ml concentrated sulfuric acid was added dropwise to the mixture. While the temperature was rose, the color of the mixture got darker. The dropping speed of concentrated sulfuric acid was controlled carefully. After that, the reaction mixture was heated to mild boiling for 60~90 min. The mixture was cooled and then poured into 80 ml of cold water, then the crude *p*-nitro benzoic acid was collected by suction filtration and washed with 45 ml water for three times. Transmitted the residue to a 100 ml beaker, and then dissolved in 76 ml warm sodium hydroxide solution (5%), and filtered a gain at about 60 ℃. After cooled down, the filtrate was poured slowly into 60 ml of 15% H_2SO_4 (aq.) with continuous stirring. The yellow color products were precipitated, filtered and washed by water. And it was dried and calculated the yield.

4.2　Preparation of ethyl-*p*-nitrobenzoate (esterification)

6 g *p*-nitro benzoic acid and 20 ml absolute ethanol were added to a 250 ml dried, round bottomed flask then 2 ml concentrated sulfuric acid was added slowly. Then the flask was equipped with a condenser with a drying tube containing calcium chloride ($CaCl_2$). Heated the mixture over water-bath to reflux for 1~1.5 h. The reaction mixture was cooled down and then poured into 85 ml water and stirred. The sodium carbonate powder was added into the mixture till the white precipitate was came out. And the 10 ml ($NaCO_3$) the solution (5%) was added into the mixture. After checked the pH, the mixture was filtered and washed with water, and dried and calculated the yield.

4.3　Synthesis of ethyl-4-aminobenzoate (reduction)

In a 100 ml three necked flask equipped with a thermometer and condenser, 6 g ethyl-*p*-nitro benzoate and 35 ml ethanol (95%), 2.5 ml acetic acid and processed iron powder 8.6 g were stirred and heated at 95~98 ℃ and refluxed for 90 min. After cooled for a few minutes, the mixture was added warm saturated solution of Na_2CO_3 fractionally (prepared by 3 g Na_2CO_3 and 30 ml H_2O) with stirring. Then the mixture filtered. The crystal precipitated was cooled, filtered and washed with diluted ethanol, and died.

4.4　Refinement

The crude product was placed in a 100 ml round bottom flask. The ethanol (50%, aq.) was added to dissolved the product by heating over water bath. After cooled down, the charcoal was added, and the mixture was refluxed for 20 min. Then the mixture was filtered. Quickly the warm filtrate was transmitted into a beaker and allowed the filtrate to cool slightly until crystals all had been precipitated. The crystals were filter and washed with a small amount of ethanol (50%, aq.) for twice. The product was dried, weighed and determined the melting point, and then calculated the yield.

4.5　Identification

4.5.1　TLC with standard substance.

4.5.2　Infrared absorption spectroscopy.

4.5.3　Nuclear magnetic resonance spectroscopy.

5. Notes

5.1   The oxidation reaction was very intense. The method of mechanical agitation and dropping sulfuric acid could make the reaction more stable and safe. After installation, the equipment should be checked by the teacher before start.

5.2   The dropping funnel should be checked before use to make sure its tightness.

5.3   If there was more white smoke or sparks in the flask when dripping with sulfuric acid, the reaction should be rapidly slowed down or suspended, and cool the flaslk with cold water is necessity.

5.4   The addition of concentrated sulfuric acid must be slow and constantly shaked, so that it is dispersed evenly in the reaction liquid, in order to prevent carbonation caused by heating.

5.5   The reaction must be vigorous shaking to emulsify the oil layer, so after cooling crystallization precipitation of fine particles, the acid was easy to remove with sodium carbonate.

5.6   *p*-nitrobenzoic acid should be added slowly due to the exothermic reaction.

5.7   The reaction must be stirred violently so that the heavy iron powder could not be deposited at the bottom of the flask.

5.8   In order to reduce the loss of products, filtration could be performed step by step.

6. Questions

6.1   Why the esterfication reaction needs anhydrous operation?

6.2   What is the mechanism of the reduction reaction?

实验五　磺胺醋酰钠的合成

一、实验目的

1. 掌握根据药物理化性质的差异分离纯化产物的方法。
2. 掌握酰化反应实验原理。
3. 进一步熟悉磺胺类药物的理化性质。

二、实验原理

磺胺醋酰钠（sulphacetamide sodium）为短效磺胺类药物，具有广谱抗菌作用，用于结膜炎、角膜炎、泪囊炎、沙眼及其他敏感菌引起的眼部感染。磺胺醋酰钠为白色结晶性粉末，无臭，微苦。易溶于水，微溶于乙醇、丙酮。化学名为 $N-$（$4-$氨基苯基）$-$磺酰基$-$乙酰胺钠一水合物，化学结构式为：

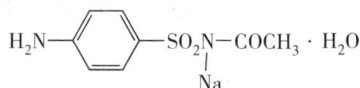

$$H_2N-\!\!\!\bigcirc\!\!\!-SO_2N-COCH_3 \cdot H_2O$$
$$\underset{Na}{|}$$

磺胺醋酰钠的合成以对氨基苯磺酰胺为原料，在碱性条件下，通过与乙酸酐在磺酰胺基 N 原子上发生乙酰化反应得到。合成路线如下：

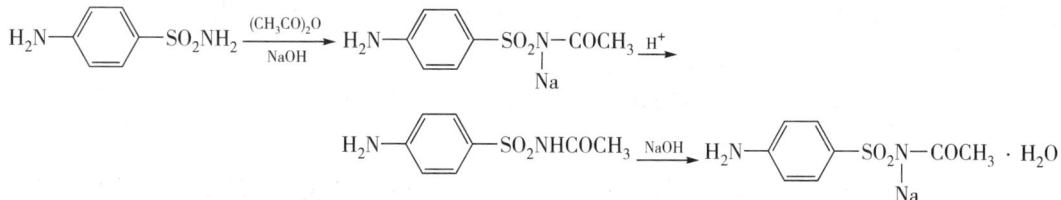

$$H_2N-\!\!\!\bigcirc\!\!\!-SO_2NH_2 \xrightarrow[NaOH]{(CH_3CO)_2O} H_2N-\!\!\!\bigcirc\!\!\!-SO_2\underset{Na}{N}-COCH_3 \xrightarrow{H^+}$$

$$H_2N-\!\!\!\bigcirc\!\!\!-SO_2NHCOCH_3 \xrightarrow{NaOH} H_2N-\!\!\!\bigcirc\!\!\!-SO_2\underset{Na}{N}-COCH_3 \cdot H_2O$$

三、仪器和试剂

仪器：磁力加热搅拌器，球形冷凝器，温度计，三颈瓶（250 ml），圆底烧瓶（100 ml），烧杯（250 ml），布氏漏斗，抽滤瓶。

试剂：磺胺，22.5% 氢氧化钠，乙酸酐，77% 的氢氧化钠，浓盐酸，10% 盐酸，40% 氢氧化钠，20% 的氢氧化钠。

四、实验步骤

（一）磺胺醋酰（SA）的制备

在装有温度计、搅拌棒和冷凝管的 100 ml 的三颈瓶中依次加入磺胺 17.2 g、22.5% 的氢氧化钠溶液 22 ml，开动搅拌器，水浴加热至 50 ℃，待物料溶解，滴加乙酸酐 3.6 ml，5

分钟后滴加 77% 的氢氧化钠溶液 2.5 ml（注 1）。此后，每隔 5 分钟交替滴加乙酸酐及 77% 的氢氧化钠溶液各 2 ml（注 2），共 5 次。加料期间反应温度维持在 50～55 ℃，保持 pH 为 12～13（注 3）。滴加完毕，保持此温度继续反应 30 分钟。反应结束，将反应液转入 100 ml 烧杯并置于冷水浴中，加入 15 ml 水，用浓盐酸调至 pH 7，室温放置 30 分钟，期间不时用玻璃棒搅拌，抽滤（注 4）。弃去固体，将所得滤液用浓盐酸调 pH 至 4～5，抽滤，弃去滤液，将所得沉淀压干（注 5）。沉淀用 3 倍量 10% 盐酸溶解，搅拌 10 分钟，抽滤，除去不溶物。滤液用 40% 氢氧化钠溶液调至 pH 5，抽滤，所得固体为磺胺醋酰（注 6）。干燥，测熔点（mp. 179～184 ℃）。如熔点不合格，可用热水（1∶15）精制。

（二）磺胺醋酰的制备

将上述制备得到的磺胺醋酰放入 50 ml 烧杯中，滴加少量水润湿（＜1 ml）（注 7）。于水浴上加热至 90 ℃，滴加 20% 的氢氧化钠至恰好溶解（注 8），此时溶液 pH 应为 7～8，室温静置，自然冷却（注 9），待析出晶体后抽滤，得磺胺醋酰钠，红外灯下干燥，称重，计算产率。

五、注意事项

1. 本实验中使用的氢氧化钠溶液有多种不同的浓度，在实验中切勿错用错配，否则会导致实验失败。

2. 滴加醋酐和氢氧化钠溶液是交替进行的，每滴完一种溶液后，再滴入另一种溶液。用玻璃吸管加入，滴加速度以每秒 2～3 滴为宜。

3. 反应液保持 pH 12～13 很重要，否则收率将会降低。

4. pH 7 时析出的固体不是产物，应弃去。产物在滤液中，切勿搞错。

5. pH 4～5 时析出的固体是产物。

6. 本实验中，溶液 pH 的调节是反应能否成功的关键，注意控制 pH 值，否则实验会失败或收率降低。

7. 加入水的量使磺胺醋酰略湿即可。可适当多加一些（1 ml 左右），在析晶时再蒸发去一些水分。

8. 磺胺醋酰制成钠盐时，按下述反应方程式计算所需 NaOH 的量，然后将其配成 20% 的 NaOH 溶液，滴加到磺胺醋酰中，切勿过量。

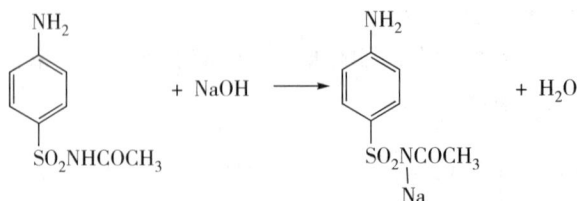

$$\text{对位—}C_6H_4(NH_2)(SO_2NHCOCH_3) + NaOH \longrightarrow \text{对位—}C_6H_4(NH_2)(SO_2N(Na)COCH_3) + H_2O$$

9. 若滤液放置后较难析出结晶，可置电炉上略加热，使其挥发去一些水分后再放冷析晶。

10. 磺胺醋酰钠的制备及去除杂质过程如图 4–1 所示。

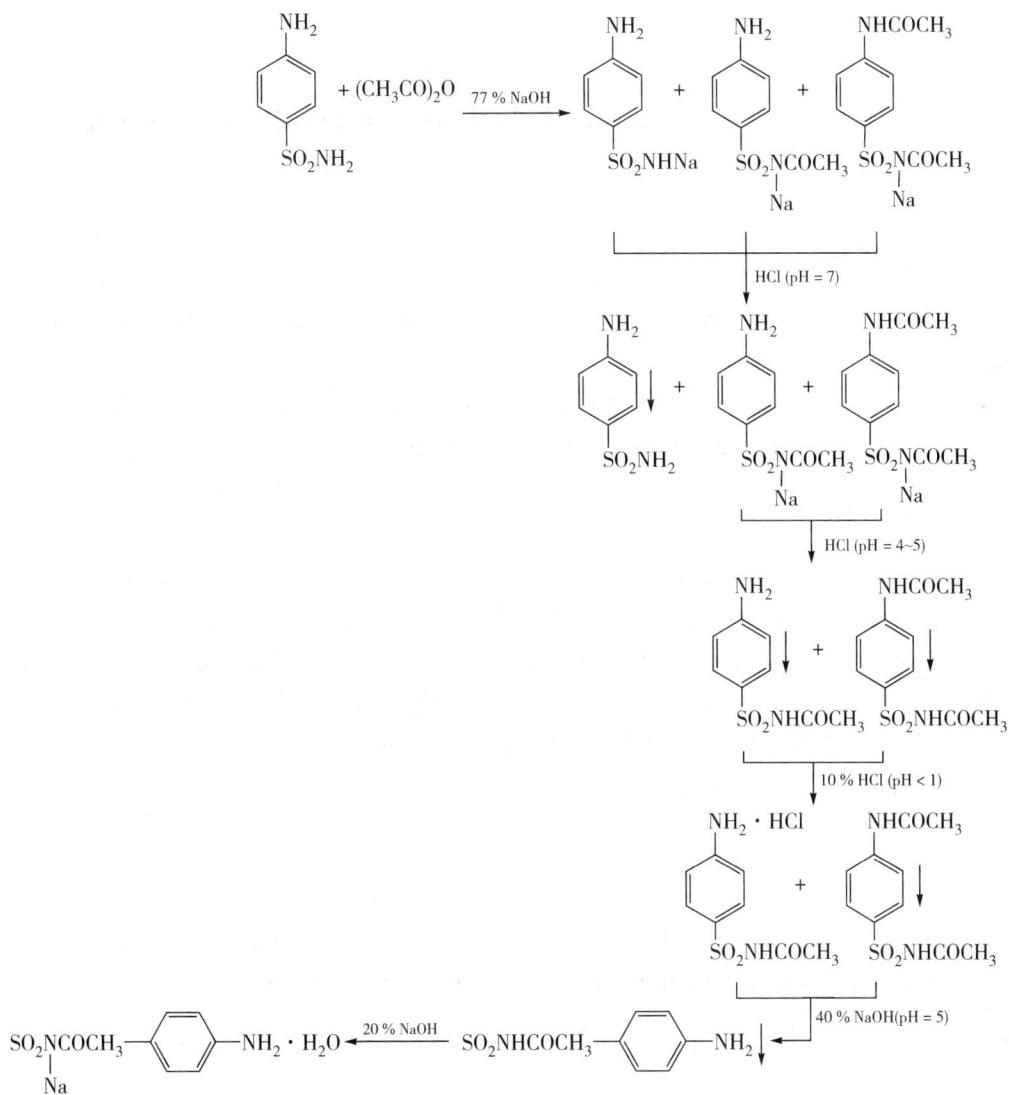

图 4－1 磺胺醋酰钠的制备及去除杂质过程示意图

六、思考

1. 磺胺类药物有哪些理化性质？本实验是如何利用这些性质进行产品纯化的？

2. 反应液处理时，pH 7 时析出的固体是什么？pH 5 时析出的固体是什么？在 10% 盐酸中的不溶物是什么？为什么？

3. 反应过程中，调节 pH 为 12～13 是非常重要的。若碱性过强，其结果是磺胺较多，磺胺醋酰次之，磺胺双醋酰较少；碱性过弱，其结果是磺胺双醋酰较多，磺胺醋酰次之，磺胺较少，为什么？

Experiment 5　Synthesis of Sulfacetamide Sodium

1. Objective

1.1　To master the method for purifying the products according to the properties of the compounds.

1.2　To master the principle and the operation of acylation reaction.

1.3　To further understand the properties of sulfanilamides.

2. Principle

Sulphacetamide sodium is a short-acting sulfonamide with antibacterial activity. It is used for curing eye infections caused by susceptible strains such as conjunctivitis, keratitis, dacryocystitis and trachoma. Sulphacetamide sodium is an odorless, slightly bitter, white crystalline powder. Freely soluble in water and slightly soluble in ethanol and acetone. The chemical name is N-[(4-aminophenyl)-sulfonyl] acetamide sodium salt monohydrate, and the structural formula is as following:

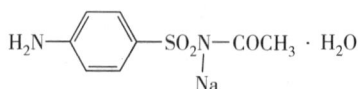

$$H_2N-\underset{}{\bigcirc}-SO_2\underset{\underset{Na}{|}}{N}-COCH_3 \cdot H_2O$$

Sulphacetamide sodium is prepared by the reaction of p-aminobenzene sulfonamide with acetic anhydride under base condition. The synthetic route is as follows:

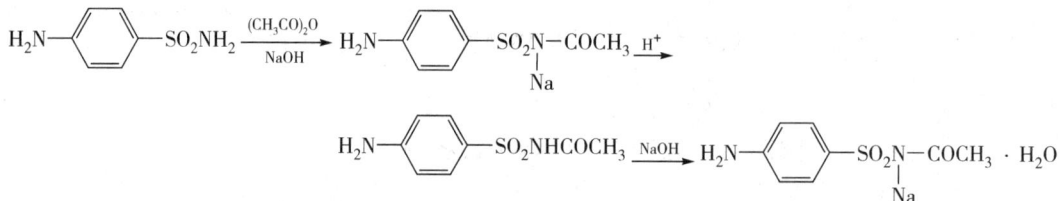

$$H_2N-\bigcirc-SO_2NH_2 \xrightarrow[NaOH]{(CH_3CO)_2O} H_2N-\bigcirc-SO_2\underset{\underset{Na}{|}}{N}-COCH_3 \xrightarrow{H^+}$$

$$H_2N-\bigcirc-SO_2NHCOCH_3 \xrightarrow{NaOH} H_2N-\bigcirc-SO_2\underset{\underset{Na}{|}}{N}-COCH_3 \cdot H_2O$$

3. Apparatus and Materials

Apparatus： magnetic heating stirrer, condenser-Allihn type, thermometer, three necked flask (250 ml), round bottom flask (100 ml), beaker (250 ml), Busher funnel, suction flask.

Materials： ulfanilamide, concentrated hydrochloric acid, sodium hydroxide aqueous solution (22.5%), sodium hydroxide aqueous solution (77%), 40% sodium hydroxide aqueous solution,

4. Procedures

4.1　The preparation of sulfacetamide (SA)

Place 17.2 g sulfanilamide and 22 ml sodium hydroxide aqueous solution (22.5%) to a 100 ml three necked flask equipped with a thermometer and reflux condenser. The reaction mixture is stirred and heated to 50 ℃ in a water bath. After the solid dissolves completely, 3.6 ml acetic anhydride and 12.5 ml sodium hydroxide aqueous solution (77%) are added dropwise to the solvent. After 5 min, 2 ml acetic anhydride and 2 ml sodium hydroxide aqueous solution (77%) are added (Note 5.1). Sequently, the same operation repeats 5 times (Note 5.2). Meanwhile, pH of the solution is kept between 12 and 13 (Note 5.3) and the temperature should be maintained between 50 to 55 ℃. After another 30 min reaction at 50~55 ℃, the reaction mixture is poured into a 100 ml beaker with an ice bath and 15 ml water. The pH of the solution is adjusted to 7 with concentrated hydrochloric acid, left to stand still for 30 min, stirred frequently.

After the reaction, collect the filtrate after suction filtration (Note 5.4). Adjust the pH to 4~5 with concentrated hydrochloric acid again, filtrate, discard the filtrate and press the precipitate as dry as possible. The solid is collected (Note 5.5). Put The solid into a beaker, dissolve it with 3 times of 10% hydrochloric acid for 10 min, then discard the undissolved substance. The filtering liquid obtained is adjusted to pH 5 with 40% sodium hydroxide aqueous solution. Sulfacetamide precipitate from the solution is collected by suction filtration (Note 5.6). Dry the product, then determine the melting point (mp. 179~184 ℃) (Note 5.7).

4.2　The preparation of sulfacetamide sodium

Put the obtained sulfacetamide into a 50 ml beater, wet it by a little water (< 1 ml) (Note 5.8), then heat to 90 ℃ in a water bath. Add calculated sodium hydroxide aqueous solution (v/v, 20%) to dissolve the sulfacetamide (Note 5.9). The pH of the solution should be between 7~8, then stand still and cool to room temperature (Note 5.10). The resultant crystal is filtrated and exposed to a infrared light. The dried sulfacetamide sodium is obtained and weighted to calculate the yield.

5. Notes

5.1　In the experiment, several different concentrations of sodium hydroxide aqueous solution are used. Careful operation is necessary; otherwise the experiment will be unsuccessful.

5.2　Acetic anhydride and 77% sodium hydroxide aqueous solution should be added every 5 min alternately. The solution should be added drop by drop.

5.3　It is important to keep the pH of the solution between 12 and 13, otherwise the yield will be lower.

5.4　The solid precipitated at pH 7 is not the product. It is unreacted sulfanilamide. The product exists in the filtrate.

5.5　The solid is a sulfacetamide when pH 4~5.

5.6　During this experiment, it is important to adjust the pH of the solution carefully. Otherwise the reaction will be failure.

5.7　Be sure not to add too much water, 1 ml water is acceptable to just wet sulfacetamide.

Extra water could be evaporated during crystal formation process if necessary.

5.8　Be sure not to add too much sodium hydroxide to sulfacetamide, just add calculated sodium hydroxide aqueous according the following reaction formula.

5.9　If no solid come out after cooled to room temperature, the solution in the beaker should be heated to remove some water, then the solid may come out after the solution is cooled.

5.10　Rout for synthesis and purification of sulfacetamide sodium (Fig. 4 − 1).

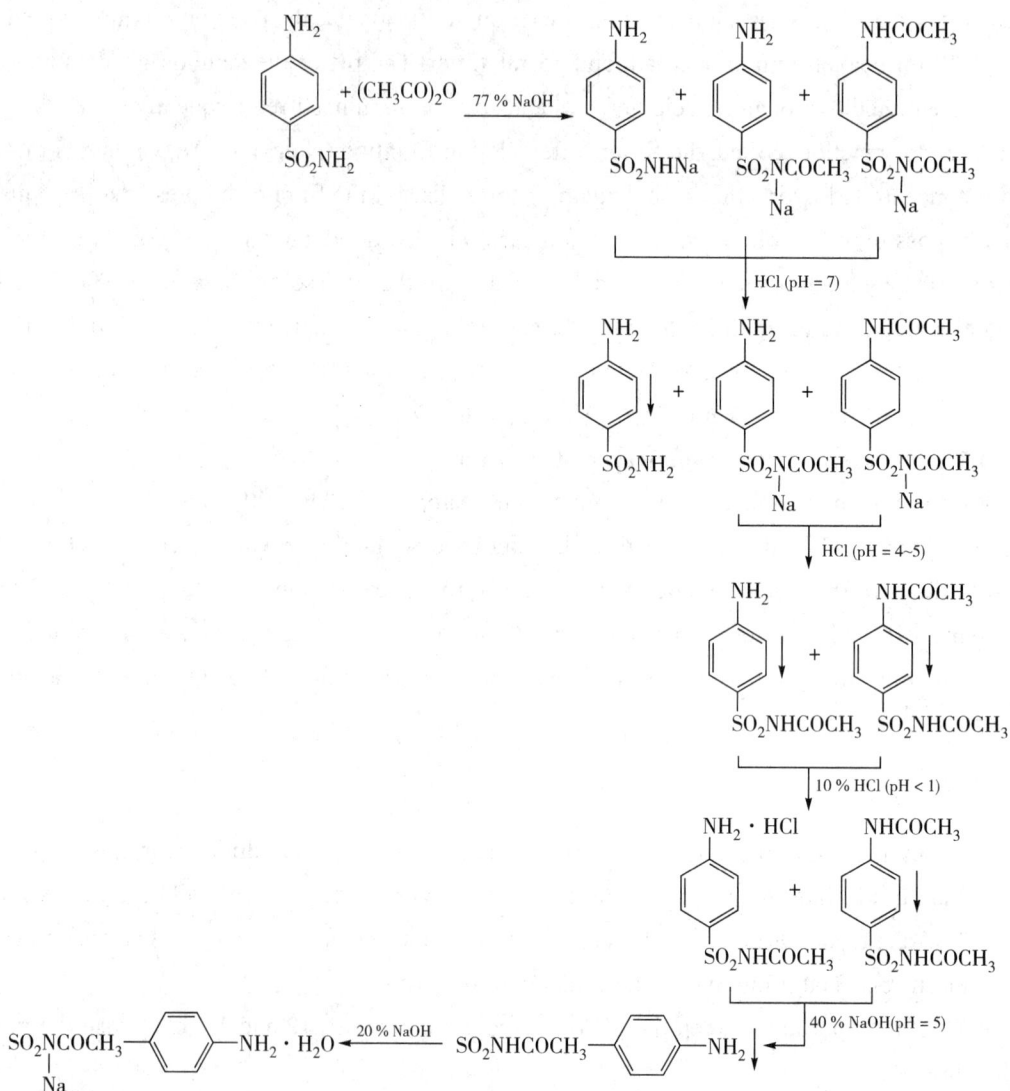

Fig. 4 − 1　Rout for synthesis and purification of sulfacetamide sodium

6. Questions

6.1　What are the physical and chemical properties of sulfacetamides? How to purify the compound based on these features?

6.2 During the reaction, what is the solid obtained at pH 7 and pH 5 respectively? What is the undissolved solid in 10% hydrochloric acid?

6.3 It is important to keep the pH of the solution between 12 and 13. What will the results be if the pH of the solution is more basic or less basic?

实验六　巴比妥的合成

一、实验目的

1. 通过对巴比妥的合成，了解药物合成的基本流程。
2. 掌握无水操作技术。

二、实验原理

巴比妥作为一种长时效的镇静催眠类药物，主要用于治疗因神经过度兴奋、狂躁或忧虑引起的失眠。巴比妥的化学名为 5，5 - 二乙基巴比妥酸，其化学结构式如下：

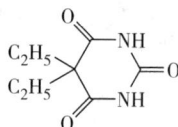

巴比妥是无臭、味略苦的白色针状结晶或结晶性粉末，熔点为 189～192 ℃。其易溶于沸水及乙醇溶剂，难溶于水，可溶于三氯甲烷、乙醚和丙酮。

通过如下合成路线，可以进行巴比妥的制备：

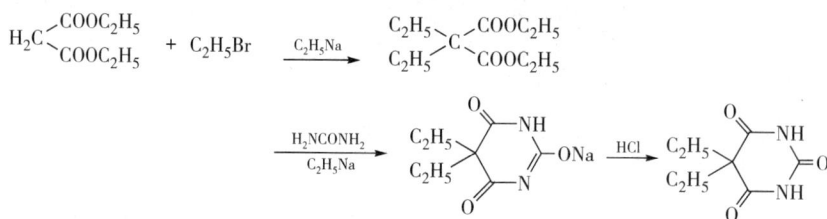

三、仪器和试剂

仪器：磁力加热搅拌器，球形冷凝器，温度计，三颈瓶（250 ml），圆底烧瓶（100 ml），烧杯（250 ml），锥形瓶，布氏漏斗，抽滤瓶。

试剂：金属钠，邻苯二甲酸二乙酯，无水乙醇，丙二酸二乙酯，溴乙烷，乙醚，尿素，活性炭，乙醇，10% $FeCl_3$ 溶液。

四、实验步骤

（一）绝对乙醇的制备

在已装有球形冷凝器(顶端配备盛有氯化钙的干燥管)的 250 ml 圆底烧瓶中加入 180 ml 的无水乙醇，添加几粒沸石，并分批加入 2 g 金属钠后，加热并回流 30 分钟；然后，加入 6 ml 的邻苯二甲酸二乙酯，并再次回流 10 分钟。待回流结束，将实验装置由回流装置改为蒸馏装置，进行蒸馏，并舍去前馏分。然后，以干燥、磨口的锥形瓶做接受器，并蒸馏至近乎无液滴流出为止。量取接受器中所收集馏分的体积，并进行密封贮存。

验证乙醇中水分的有无，通常的检验方法是：在一支干燥的试管中，加入 1 ml 已制得的绝对乙醇，并立即加入少量无水硫酸铜粉末。如果试管中的无水硫酸铜变为蓝色，则说明制得的绝对乙醇中含有水分。

（二）二乙基丙二酸二乙酯的制备

在装有温度计、滴液漏斗及球形冷凝器（顶端附有氯化钙干燥管）的 250 ml 三颈瓶中，加入 75 ml 上述制备的绝对乙醇，并分批加入 6 g 金属钠。待反应缓慢时，开始搅拌，油浴加热（油浴温度不超过 90 ℃）。待反应器中金属钠消失后，利用滴液漏斗向其内加入 18 ml 丙二酸二乙酯（10～15 分钟内完成），并回流反应 15 分钟。待反应体系的温度降至低于 50 ℃ 时，缓慢滴加 20 ml 溴乙烷（约 15 分钟加完），并继续回流反应 2.5 小时。待反应结束，将实验装置由回流装置改为蒸馏装置，进行乙醇的蒸除（但不要蒸干）。完成后，放置冷却，药渣用 40～45 ml 的水溶解，并转移到分液漏斗中，分取酯层；水层用乙醚萃取 3 次（20 ml 乙醚/每次），合并酯层与醚提取液，并用 20 ml 水再洗涤一次，分取有机相并倒入 150 ml 的锥形瓶中，加入 5 g 无水硫酸钠干燥，密封放置。

（三）二乙基丙二酸二乙酯的蒸馏

将步骤二制得的二乙基丙二酸二乙酯乙醚液过滤，收集滤液并蒸除乙醚。瓶内的剩余液，用装有空气冷凝管的蒸馏装置于砂浴上蒸馏，并用预先称量的 50 ml 锥形瓶收集 218～222 ℃馏分，称重，计算收率，密封保存。

（四）巴比妥的制备

在装有搅拌子、温度计及球型冷凝器（顶端附有氯化钙干燥管）的 250 ml 三颈瓶中加入 50 ml 乙醇，并分次加入 2.6 g 金属钠，待反应缓慢时，开始搅拌。待金属钠消失后，分别加入 10 g 二乙基丙二酸二乙酯、4.4 g 尿素。加入完成后，随即使内温升高至 80～82 ℃，停止搅拌，并保温反应 80 分钟（正常反应时，停止搅拌 5～10 分钟后，料液中会有小气泡逸出，并逐渐呈微沸状态，有时较激烈）。反应完成后，将回流装置改为蒸馏装置。在搅拌条件下慢慢蒸除乙醇，直至常压不易蒸出时，再减压蒸馏尽。残渣用 80 ml 水溶解，并转移至盛有 18 ml 稀盐酸（盐酸:水 = 1:1）的 250 ml 烧杯中，调 pH 3～4，结晶析出，抽滤，得粗品。

（五）巴比妥的精制

粗品称重后，置于 150 ml 的锥形瓶中，用水（16 ml/g）加热使溶解，加入少许活性炭，脱色反应 15 分钟，并趁热抽滤。待滤液冷至室温，即析出白色结晶产物，抽滤，水洗，烘干，计算收率，测熔点。

五、注意事项

1. 本实验所用仪器均需彻底干燥。考虑到无水乙醇具有很强的吸水性，因此在操作及存放时，必须防止水分的侵入。

2. 无水乙醇作为制备绝对乙醇的前驱体，其内水分含量不能超过 0.5%，否则反应不容易进行。

3. 在用镊子进行金属钠取用时，先用滤纸吸去沾附在金属钠上的油，并用小刀切去其表面的氧化层后，再切成小块。切下来的钠屑应放回原瓶中，切忌与滤纸一起投入废物缸中，并严禁与水接触，以免引起燃烧爆炸事故。

4. 邻苯二甲酸二乙酯的加入，可以和氢氧化钠进行如下反应：

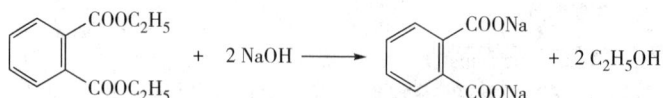

$$\text{邻苯二甲酸二乙酯（COOC}_2\text{H}_5\text{、COOC}_2\text{H}_5\text{)} + 2\text{NaOH} \longrightarrow \text{邻苯二甲酸二钠（COONa、COONa)} + 2\text{C}_2\text{H}_5\text{OH}$$

因此，可以避免乙醇与氢氧化钠生成的乙醇钠再和水发生作用，从而可以使制得的乙醇达到极高的纯度。

5. 溴乙烷的沸点很低，用量也要随室温而变。当室温在 30 ℃ 左右时，应加溴乙烷 28 ml，同时滴加溴乙烷所用的时间应适当延长；若室温在 30 ℃ 以下，可按本实验方案投料。

6. 待反应体系温度降到 50 ℃，再慢慢滴加溴乙烷，以避免溴乙烷的挥发及生成乙醚的副反应。

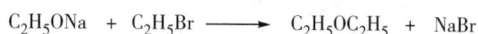

$$\text{C}_2\text{H}_5\text{ONa} + \text{C}_2\text{H}_5\text{Br} \longrightarrow \text{C}_2\text{H}_5\text{OC}_2\text{H}_5 + \text{NaBr}$$

7. 由于砂浴传热慢，因此砂要铺得薄，也可采用减压蒸馏的方法。

8. 尿素需在 60 ℃ 提前干燥 4 小时。

9. 蒸乙醇速度不宜快，至少要用 80 分钟，反应才能顺利进行。

六、思考

1. 在进行无水试剂的制备时应注意什么问题？为什么在进行加热回流和蒸馏时冷凝管的顶端和接受器的支管上都要装置盛有氯化钙的干燥管？

2. 工业上如何制备无水乙醇（99.5%）？

3. 通常如何对液体产物进行精制？本实验用水洗涤提取液的目的是什么？

Experiment 6 Synthesis of Barbital

1. Objective

1.1 To understand the fundamental process in drug synthesis via the synthesis of barbital.

1.2 To grasp the anhydrous operation.

2. Principle

As a long-acting sedative-hypnotic drug, barbital is mainly used to treat insomnia caused by over-excitation, mania or anxiety. The chemical name of barbital is 5,5-diethylbarbituric acid, whose chemical structure is as follows:

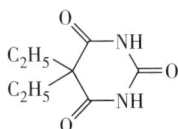

Barbitalis odorless, slightly bitter white needle-like crystalline or crystalline powder with a melting point of $189 \sim 192 \, ^\circ\!C$. It is soluble in boiling water and ethanol solvent, while insoluble in water, and soluble in chloroform, diethylether and acetone.

Barbital can be prepared by the following synthetic route:

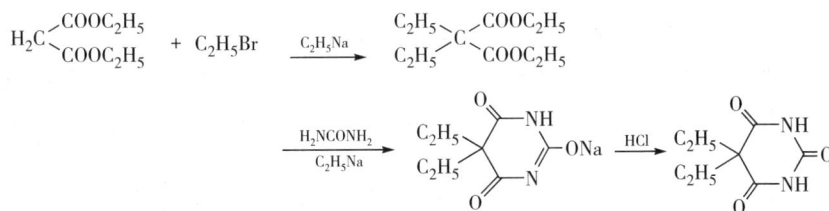

3. Apparatus and Materials

Apparatus: magnetic heating stirrer, condenser-Allihn type, thermometer, three necked flask (250 ml), round bottom flask (100 ml), beaker (250 ml), beakerflask, Busher funnel, suction flask.

Materials: anhydrous ethanol, sodium, diethyl phthalate, diethyl malonate, ethyl bromide, diethyl ether, urea, activated carbon.

4. Procedures

4.1 Synthesis of absolute ethanol

180 ml anhydrous ethanol and several pieces of zeolite were added to a 250 ml round

bottom flask equipped with a round condenser (a dry tube containing calcium chloride equipped at the top), then followed by 2 g of sodium and refluxed for 30 min.Then, 6 ml of diethyl phthalate was added and refluxed again for 10 min. At the end of the reflux, the experimental device was switched from the reflux device into a distillation unit, and discarding the fore distillate.Then, a dry ground flask was used as a receiver and distilled until almost no droplets ran out. Measure the volume of the collection in the receiver and seal them for storage.

The general method to verify the presence of water in ethanol: add 1 ml of absolute ethanol to a dry test tube, and then immediately followed by a small amount of anhydrous copper sulfate powder.If the anhydrous copper sulfate would turn to blue, then the produced absolute ethanol contains moisture.

4.2　Synthesis of ethyl diethylmalonate

75 ml of absolute ethanol prepared above was added to a 250 ml three-necked flask equipped with a thermometer, dropping funnel and a round condenser (a drying tube filled with calcium chloride equipped at the top), and then followed by 6 g of sodium metal in portions. When the reaction is slow, start agitation and heat it in an oil bath (oil bath temperature should not exceed 90 ℃).After the disappearance of sodium in the reactor, 18 ml of diethyl malonate was added dropwise by the dropping funnel within 10～15 min, and refluxed for 15 min.When the temperature of the reaction system dropped below 50 ℃, 20 ml of ethyl bromide was added slowly within 15 min and refluxed for 2.5 h.When the reaction is over, change the experimental device from the reflux device to the distillation device and perform the ethanol evaporation (but do not evaporate to dryness).After cooled, the residue was dissolved by 40～45 ml of water, and then transferred to a separating funnel to separate the ester layer. The water layer was extracted with diethyl ether (20 ml per time) for three times. Then combined ester layers and ether extracts together, and wash the combined extract with another 20 ml of water. Next, the organic phase was collected and transferred into a 150 ml conical flask, and dried over 5 g of anhydrous sodium sulfate.

4.3　Distillation of ethyl diethylmalonate

Filtrate the diethyl diethylmalonate diethyl ether obtained in Step 4.2, and distill off the ether. The residue was distilled at a sand bath using a distillation apparatus equipped with an air-cooled condenser, and distillation ranging from 218 to 222 ℃ were collected by using a pre-weighed 50 ml conical flask, weight and calculate the yield. The corresponding product was sealed and deposited.

4.4　Synthesis of Barbital

50 ml of absolute ethanol was added to a 250 ml three-necked flask equipped with a stirrer, a thermometer and a round condenser(equipped with a dry tube filled with calcium chloride at the top), then followed by 2.6 g sodium in batches. When the reaction was slow, starting to stir.After the metal sodium disappeared, 10 g of diethyl diethylmalonate and 4.4 g of urea were added,respectively.After the addition is complete, the reactants were heated to 80～82 ℃. Then,

stop stirring and incubate the reaction for 80 min (normally, small bubbles will escape from the solvent after stopping stirring for 5～10 min. Then the whole reactants turned boiling and sometimes even more drastic). Then, the reflux device was changed to a distillation unit.Evaporate the ethanol slowly with stirring and distilled off under reduced pressure until the ethanol could not be evaporated under the general pressure.The residue was dissolved by 80 ml of water and transferred to a 250 ml beaker. The pH value was adjusted between 3 and 4 by using diluted hydrochloric acid (hydrochloric acid:water = 1:1), the resulting crystals were filtered and obtaining the crude product.

4.5　Refinement of Barbital

The crude product was weighed and placed in a 150 ml conical flask, heated to dissolve it with water (16 ml / g), and then, added a little activated carbon and decolo red for 15 min and filtered while hot.When the filtrate was cooled to room temperature, a white crystalline product was produced, and then filtrate, and the product was washed by water, dried, calculated the yield and measured the melting point.

5. Notes

5.1　The instruments used in this experiment are needed to be dried thoroughly. Considering the anhydrous ethanol has a strong water absorption, you must prevent the invasion of moisture during operation and storage.

5.2　Anhydrous ethanol is the precursor for the preparation of absolute ethanol, its water content cannot exceed 0.5%, and otherwise the reaction is not easy to carry out.

5.3　A forceps is used in fetching the sodium, firstly with the filter paper to absorb the adhered oil, secondly cut the oxide layer on the surface of sodium with a knife, and then cut the sodium into small pieces.The waste sodium must be returned to the original bottle,should not be thrown away into a waste bin together with filter papers. Additionally, sodium is not allowed to contact with water to avoid explosion accidents.

5.4　Diethyl phthal ateadded in the system can react with hydroxyl sodium as follows:

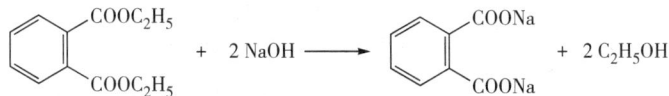

Therefore, sodium ethylated, produced by ethanol and sodium hydroxide can be prevented from reacting with water again, and the purity of the prepared ethanol can be extremely high.

5.5　Ethyl bromidehas a very low boiling point and its dosage will be varied with room temperature. When the room temperature is about 30 ℃, 28 ml of ethyl bromide should be added, and the correspond time for the dropwise addition should be extended; If the room temperature is below 30 ℃, it could be operated according to the aforementioned experimental program.

5.6　Ethyl bromide would not be dropped until the temperature of the reaction system fell down to 50 ℃, which will avoid the volatilization of ethyl bromide and side reactions to produce diethyl ether.

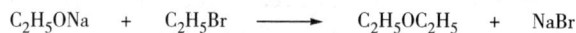

$$C_2H_5ONa \ + \ C_2H_5Br \ \longrightarrow \ C_2H_5OC_2H_5 \ + \ NaBr$$

5.7 Due to the slow diathermanous rate of sand bath, a thin layer of sand is need. Alternatively, a distillation under reduced pressure could also be used.

5.8 The urea must be pre-dried at 60 ℃ for 4 h.

5.9 The speed for ethanol evaporation should not be fast, and 80 min is needed at least, thus the reaction can be carried out smoothly.

6. Questions

6.1 What attention should be paid to during the preparation of absolute ethanol? Why a tube filled with calcium chloride must be equipped at the top of the condenser and the side pipe of the receptor during a process of reflux and distillation?

6.2 How to produce absolute ethanol (99.5%) in industry?

6.3 Generally, how to refine the liquid product? What is the purpose of washing the extracts with water in this experiment?

实验七　扁桃酸的合成

一、实验目的

1. 熟悉相转移催化反应机制、卡宾反应机制。
2. 通过扁桃酸的合成，掌握药物合成的基本操作技术。

二、实验原理

扁桃酸，又名苦杏仁酸、α-羟基苯乙酸，是有机合成的重要中间体，也是口服治疗尿道感染的药物。扁桃酸结构中有一个不对称碳原子，化学合成方法得到的是外消旋体，旋光性的碱如麻黄素可将其拆分为单一异构体。

扁桃酸传统上可用扁桃腈［$C_6H_5CH(OH)CN$］和 α,α-二氯苯乙酮（$C_6H_5COCHCl_2$）的水解来制备，但合成路线长、操作繁琐且具危险。本实验采用相转移催化（PT）法，只需一步反应即可得到产物。反应路线如下：

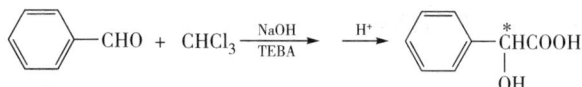

一般认为反应机制是反应中产生的二氯卡宾对苯甲醛的羰基加成，再经重排及水解制得产物。

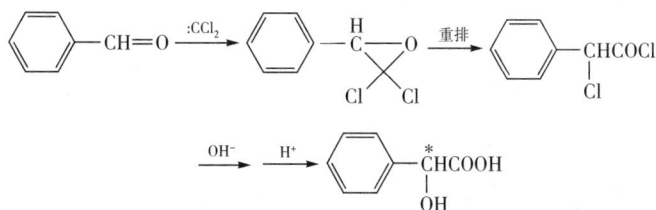

三、仪器和试剂

仪器：磁力加热搅拌器，球形冷凝器，温度计，三颈瓶（250 ml），锥形瓶，圆底烧瓶（100 ml），烧杯（250 ml），布氏漏斗，抽滤瓶。

试剂：氢氧化钠，苯甲醛，TEBA（苄基三乙基氯化铵），三氯甲烷，50%氢氧化钠溶液，乙酸乙酯，50%硫酸，甲苯，无水乙醇，石油醚。

四、实验步骤

取 250 ml 锥形瓶，加入 13 ml 水，分两次将 13 g 氢氧化钠溶于其中，搅拌冷却至室温。向装有搅拌子、冷凝管和温度计的 250 ml 三颈瓶中，加入 6.8 ml 苯甲醛、0.7 g TEBA（苄基三乙基氯化铵）和 12 ml 三氯甲烷，油浴加热，待温度上升至 50～60 ℃时，自滴液漏斗缓缓滴加配制的 50% 的氢氧化钠溶液，滴加过程中控制反应温度在 60～65 ℃，滴加完毕，再继续保持此温度搅拌反应 1 小时（注 1）。

反应混合物冷却至室温，在反应混合物中加入 140 ml 水，倒入分液漏斗中，除去下层三氯甲烷层，每次用 20 ml 乙酸乙酯萃取两次，合并乙酸乙酯层萃取液，倒入指定容器待回收乙酸乙酯。将亮黄色透明状的水层用 50% 硫酸酸化至 pH 为 1～2 后，再每次用 30 ml 乙酸乙酯萃取两次，合并酸化后的乙酸乙酯层萃取液，用无水硫酸钠干燥、过夜。

油浴中常压蒸馏除去乙酸乙酯，得粗产物。

将粗产物用甲苯–无水乙醇（注 2）（8:1，v/v）进行重结晶（每克粗产物约需 3 ml），趁热过滤，母液在室温下放置，结晶慢慢析出。冷却后抽滤，并用少量石油醚（30～60 ℃）洗涤促使其快干。产品为白色结晶，干燥，称重，计算收率（产物，mp. 118～119 ℃）。

五、注意事项

1. 此时可取反应液用试纸测其 pH，应接近中性，否则可适当延长反应时间。
2. 也可单独用甲苯重结晶。

六、思考

1. 酸化前后两次用乙酸乙酯萃取的目的何在？
2. 实验过程中为什么必须保持充分的搅拌？

Experiment 7　Synthesis of Mandelic acid

1. Objective

1.1　Be familiar with the mechanism of phase transfer catalytic reaction and carbene reaction.

1.2　To master the basic process of drug synthesis through the synthesis of mandelic acid.

2. Principle

Mandelic acid, amygdalic acid, α-hydroxyphenylacetic acid, is an important organic intermediate and can also be used as an oral therapy in treatment of urinary tract infections. Racemate was obtained through chemical synthesis for it contains a chiral carbon atom. Chiral separation of racemate could be achieved by using the chiral molecules such as ephedrine.

Mandelic acid was traditionally prepared by the hydrolysis of mandelic acid nitrile or dichlorobenzenethanone, but the synthetic route is long and the operation is difficult and of less safety. Herein the phase transfer catalysis was used and the product could be obtained in one step reaction.

The synthetic route is as follow:

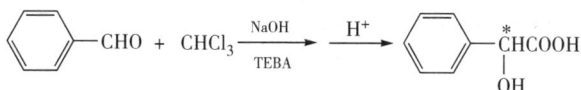

The supposed mechanism was the dichlorocarbene produced in the reaction worked with benzaldehyde through the carbonyl addition reaction, and then following rearrangement and hydrolysis to get the product.

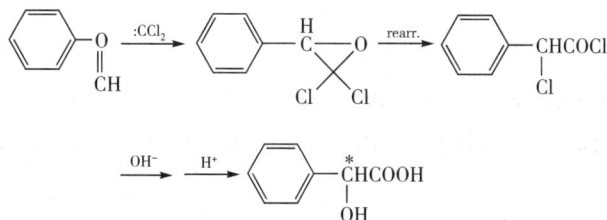

3. Apparatus and Materials

Apparatus: magnetic heating stirrer, condenser-Allihn type, thermometer, three necked flask (250 ml), beaker flask, round bottom flask (100 ml), beaker (250 ml), Busher funnel, suction flask.

Materials: Sodium hydroxide, benzaldehyde, benzyl triethylammonium chloride, chloroform,

45

50% sodium hydroxide aq., ethyl acetate, 50% H$_2$SO$_4$, toluene, anhydrous ethanol.

4. Procedures

Sodium hydroxide aqueous solution (13 g in 13 ml H$_2$O) was carefully prepared in beaker flask and then cooled and stirred to room temperature.

Benzaldehyde (6.8 ml) was added to a 250 ml three necked flask equipped with stirrer, drop funnel and thermometer, then followed by 0.7 g TEBA (benzyl triethylammonium chloride) and chloroform (12 ml). The reactant was stirred on an oil bath and when the temperature arrived 50~60 ℃, 50% sodium hydroxide aq. was added dropwise through the funnel and the temperature was controlled between 60~65 ℃. The reaction mixture was kept in this temperature for 1 hr (Note 5.1).

The residue was diluted with H$_2$O (140 ml) and extracted with ethyl acetate (20 ml per time), the combined ethyl acetate phase was poured into the container. The yellow and clear water phase was adjusted the pH to 1~2 using 50% H$_2$SO$_4$, then extracted with ethyl acetate (30 ml per time). The combined ethyl acetate phase was dried over anhydrous sodium sulfate and then the ethyl acetate was removed on oil bath and following evaporation to get the crude.

The crude was recrystallized by the mixed toluene and anhydrous ethanol (v:v=8:1, 3 ml solvent for 1 g crude) (Note 5.2). Filtrated while the solvent was hot, cooled the filtrate naturally at room temperature and then with ice bath to complete the crystallization. Filtrate and washed with petroleum ether (30~60 ℃). Dried and the mandelic acid was obtained in white crystal (mp.118~119 ℃). Weighed, calculated yield.

5. Notes

5.1   pH of the reaction should be neutral from test paper, otherwise the reaction time can be prolonged.

5.2   Toluene can be used alone for the crystallization.

6. Questions

6.1   What is the purpose of using ethyl acetate for the extraction twice in the experiment?

6.2   Why the reaction should be continued stirred during the experiment?

实验八　乙酰苯胺的制备

一、实验目的

1. 熟悉酰化反应及酰化试剂的特点。
2. 掌握回流和重结晶的操作技术。

二、实验原理

乙酰苯胺是有机合成反应中重要的有机中间体,本身亦具有很好的退热作用,俗称"退热冰",但因其毒副作用较大不能作为药物使用,临床上用其类似物作为解热镇痛药物。

乙酰苯胺由苯胺和乙酸酐在锌粉催化下发生酰化反应制得,化学反应式如下:

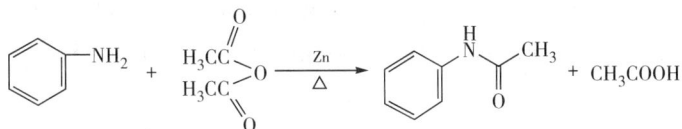

乙酰苯胺为一白色片状结晶,mp.114 ℃,不溶于冷水,微溶于热水,可用热水重结晶。

三、仪器和试剂

仪器:磁力加热搅拌器,球形冷凝器,温度计,三颈瓶(250 ml),圆底烧瓶(100 ml),烧杯(250 ml),布氏漏斗,抽滤瓶。

试剂:苯胺,乙酸酐,锌粉,活性炭。

四、实验步骤

6 ml 苯胺(6.2 g,0.66 mol),10 ml 乙酸酐(10.6 g,0.1 mol)和少量锌粉(约 0.2 g)加入到配有温度计、冷凝管、搅拌器的 250 ml 三颈瓶中,加热回流。30 分钟后将反应液倾入 200 ml 冷水中,冷却至沉淀析出。沉淀经减压过滤并用冷水洗涤至中性,制得乙酰苯胺粗品。

将粗品溶于 200 ml 热水中,加入 1 g 活性炭,回流 10 分钟后,冷却、过滤,得乙酰苯胺精品。待干燥后称重并计算产率。

五、思考

1. 提纯固体化合物的常用方法是什么?如何用简单的方法验证化合物的纯度?
2. 为什么粗产品可以用冷水洗至中性?

Experiment 8   Synthesis of Acetanilide

1. Objective

1.1   To be familiar with acylation reaction and the characteristics of acylation reagents.

1.2   To master the operation skills of refluxing and recrystallization.

2. Principle

Acetanilide, also named as "antipyretic ice" for its admirable antipyretic effect, is not fit for clinical treatment because of its serious side effect. However, it is an important intermediate in the synthesis of other organic compounds.

Acetanilide could be obtained through acylation reaction, in which aniline reacts with acetic anhydride by using zinc powder as catalyst.The synthetic route is as follow:

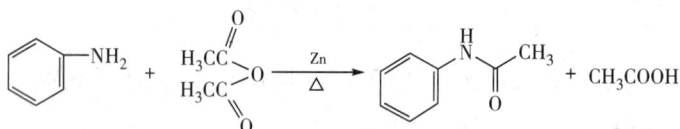

Pure acetanilide, which is a white crystalline platelet with the melting point of 114 ℃, is insoluble in cold water but could be dissolved slightly in hot water. The recrystallization of acetanilide could be carried out by using hot water as solvent.

3. Apparatus and Materials

Apparatus: magnetic heating stirrer, condenser-Allihn type, thermometer, three necked flask (250 ml), round bottom flask (100 ml), beaker (250 ml), Busher funnel, suction flask.

Materials: aniline, acetic anhydride, zinc powder, active carbon.

4. Procedures

Add 6 ml of aniline (6.2 g, 0.66 mol), 10 ml of acetic anhydride (10.6 g, 0.1 mol) and a bit of zinc powder (about 0.2 g) in a three-neck flask (250 ml) equipped with a stirrer, a thermometer and a condenser. After refluxing for 30 minutes, the hot reaction mixture is poured into 200 ml of cold water. The crude product will crystallize out. Then the crude product is collected by filtering the suspension through a decompression filtration apparatus. Wash the crystals with cold water until it is free from acid.

The crude acetanilide and about 1 g of active carbon are added in 200 ml of hot water together. After refluxing for 10 minutes, the mixture is cooled and filtered. The fine acetanilide could be obtained. The yield of acetanilide could then be calculated after drying.

5. Questions

5.1　Try to write down some most commonly used methods to purify solid organic compounds. How to identify the purification of acetanilide with a simple method?

5.2　In this experiment, the crude product could be washed to neutral using cold water, why?

实验九 诺氟沙星的合成

一、实验目的

1. 通过合成诺氟沙星，掌握药物合成的基本操作技术。
2. 通过对诺氟沙星合成路线比较，掌握选择实际生产工艺的基本要求。
3. 掌握各步中间体的质量控制方法。

二、实验原理

诺氟沙星的化学名：1－乙基－6－氟－1, 4－二氢－4－氧代－7－（1－哌嗪基）－3－喹啉羧酸。化学结构式为：

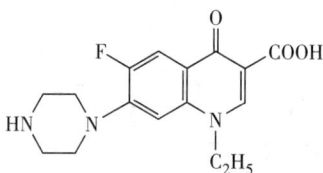

诺氟沙星为微黄色针状晶体或结晶性粉末，mp. 216~220 ℃，易溶于酸或碱，难溶于冷水。

诺氟沙星的制备方法很多，按不同原料及反应路线可分为十几条。以下为我国工业生产主要路线：

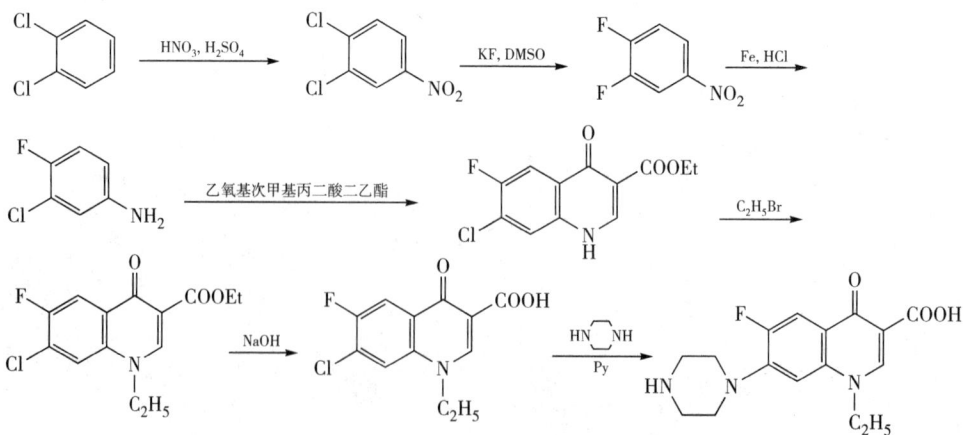

近几年来，诺氟沙星的生产出现了一些新工艺，其中硼螯合物法具有产率高、操作简便、能耗低、产品质量较好的优点：

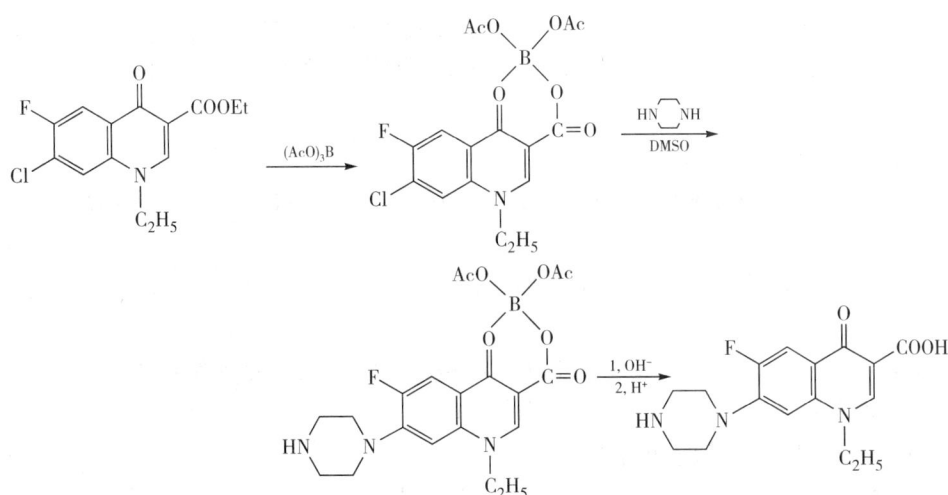

三、仪器和试剂

仪器：磁力加热搅拌器，球形冷凝器，温度计，滴液漏斗，四颈瓶（250 ml），圆底烧瓶（100 ml），烧杯（250 ml），布氏漏斗，抽滤瓶。

试剂：硝酸，浓硫酸，邻二氯苯，3,4-二氯硝基苯，二甲亚砜，氟化钾，铁粉，氯化钠，浓盐酸，原甲酸三乙酯，$ZnCl_2$，乙酸酐，无水碳酸钾，DMF，无水哌嗪，二甲亚砜。

四、实验步骤

（一）3,4-二氯硝基苯的制备

向装有搅拌器、回流冷凝器、温度计、滴液漏斗的四颈瓶中，加入硝酸 51 g，水浴冷却下，滴加浓硫酸 79 g，控制滴加速度，温度保持在 50 ℃ 以下。滴加完毕，更换滴液漏斗，于 40～50 ℃，滴加邻二氯苯 35 g，滴毕，升温至 60 ℃，反应 2 小时，静置分层，上层油状液体倾入 5 倍量水中，搅拌，固化，放置 30 分钟，过滤，水洗至 pH＝6～7，真空干燥，称重，计算产率。

注意事项

1. 本反应用混酸硝化。硫酸可防止副反应发生，并可增加被硝化物的溶解度。硝酸生成 NO_2^+，是硝化剂。

2. 发生此硝化反应，温度需达到 40 ℃，低于此温度，滴加混酸会导致大量混酸聚集，一旦反应引发，聚集的混酸会使反应温度急剧升高，发生危险，并生成大量副产物，因此，滴加混酸时应控制滴加速度，反应温度保持在 40～50 ℃。

3. 上述方法所得的产品纯度足够用于下一步反应，如需得到更纯的产品，可以采用水蒸气蒸馏法或减压蒸馏法纯化。

4. 3,4-二氯硝基苯的 mp. 39～41 ℃，不能用红外灯或烘箱干燥。

（二）4-氟-3-氯-硝基苯的合成

向装有搅拌器、回流冷凝器、温度计、氯化钙干燥管的四颈瓶中，加入 3,4-二氯硝基苯 40 g、二甲亚砜 73 g、氟化钾 23 g，回流（194～198 ℃），快速搅拌 1～1.5 小时，冷却至 50 ℃左右，加入水 75 ml，充分搅拌，倒入分液漏斗中，静置分层，分出下层油状物。安装水蒸气蒸馏装置，进行水蒸气蒸馏，得淡黄色固体，过滤，水洗至中性，真空干燥，称重，计算产率。

注意事项

1. 该步氟化反应为无水反应，所有仪器、药品及试剂必须无水，微量水会导致产率大幅下降。

2. 为保证反应液的无水状态，可在刚回流时蒸出少量二甲亚砜，将反应液中的微量水分带出。

3. 进行水蒸气蒸馏时，少量冷凝水就已足够，大量冷凝水会导致 4－氟－3－氯－硝基苯固化，堵塞冷凝管。

（三）4－氟－3－氯－苯胺的制备

向装有搅拌器、回流冷凝器、温度计的三颈瓶中，加入铁粉 51.5 g、水 173 ml、氯化钠 4.3 g、浓盐酸 2 ml，搅拌下于 100 ℃活化 10 分钟，降温至 85 ℃，快速搅拌，先加入 4－氟－3－氯－硝基苯 15 g，温度自然升至 95 ℃，10 分钟后，再加入 4－氟－3－氯－硝基苯 15 g，于 95 ℃反应 2 小时水蒸气蒸馏反应液，馏出液中加入冰，使产品固化完全，过滤，真空干燥，称重，计算产率。（产物，mp. 44～47 ℃）

注意事项

1. 胺通常是在盐酸或醋酸存在下用铁粉还原硝基化合物而制得。该法原料便宜，操作简便，产率稳定，适于工业生产。

2. 铁粉表面由于具有氧化铁膜，需经活化才能反应，铁粉粗细一般以 60 目为宜。

3. 由于铁粉密度较大，搅拌速度慢则不能将铁粉搅匀，会在烧瓶下部结块，影响产率，因此该反应应剧烈搅拌。

4. 水蒸气蒸馏应控制冷凝水的流速，防止 4－氟－3－氯－苯胺固化，堵塞冷凝管。

5. 4－氟－3－氯－苯胺的熔点低（40～43 ℃），故应低温干燥。

（四）乙氧基次甲基丙二酸二乙酯（EMME）的制备

向装有搅拌器、温度计、滴液漏斗、蒸馏装置的四颈瓶中，加入原甲酸三乙酯 78 g，$ZnCl_2$ 0.1 g，搅拌，加热，升温至 120 ℃，蒸出乙醇，降温至 70 ℃，于 70～80 ℃内再滴加原甲酸三乙酯 20 g 及醋酐 6.0 g，于 0.5 小时内滴完，然后升温到 152～156 ℃，反应 2 小时。冷却至室温，将反应液倾入圆底烧瓶中，水泵减压回收原甲酸三乙酯（bp. 140 ℃，70 ℃/5333 Pa）。冷却至室温，换油泵进行减压蒸馏，收集 120～140 ℃/666.6 Pa 的馏分，称重，计算产率。

注意事项

1. 减压蒸馏所需真空度要达 666.6 Pa 以下，才可进行蒸馏操作，真空度小，蒸馏温度高，导致产率下降。

2. 减压回收原甲酸三乙酯时亦可进行常压蒸馏，收集 140～150 ℃的沸点馏分。蒸出的原甲酸三乙酯可以重复利用。

（五）7-氯-6-氟-1，4-二氢-4-氧代喹啉-3-羧酸乙酯（环合物）的制备

向装有搅拌器、回流冷凝器、温度计的三颈瓶中，分别加入 4-氟-3-氯-苯胺 15 g、EMME 24 g，快速搅拌下加热至 120 ℃，于 120～130 ℃反应 2 h。放冷至室温，将回流装置换成蒸馏装置，加入石蜡油 80 ml，加热至 260～270 ℃，有大量乙醇生成，回收乙醇，30 分钟后，冷却至 60 ℃以下，过滤，滤饼分别用甲苯、丙酮洗至灰白色，干燥，称重，计算产率。（产物，mp. 297～298 ℃）

注意事项

1. 本反应为无水反应，所有仪器应干燥，严格按无水反应操作进行，否则会导致 EMME 分解。

2. 环合反应温度控制在 260～270 ℃，为避免温度超过 270 ℃，可在将要达到 270 ℃ 时缓慢加热。反应液变黏稠后，为避免局部过热，应快速搅拌。

3. 该环合反应为 Could-Jacobs 反应，考虑苯环上取代基的定位效应及空间效应，3-位氯的对位远比邻位活泼，但也不能忽略邻位的取代。反应条件控制不当，会生成副产物，如下式：

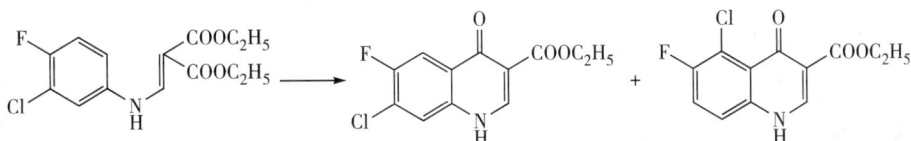

为减少反环物的生成，应注意以下几点：① 反应温度低，有利于反环物的生成。因此，反应温度应快速达到 260 ℃，且保持在 260～270 ℃。② 加大溶剂用量可以降低反环物的生成。从经济的角度来讲，采用溶剂与反应物用量比为 3:1 时比较合适。③ 用二甲苯或二苯砜为溶剂时，会减少反环物的生成，但价格昂贵。另外，可用廉价的工业柴油代替石蜡油。

（六）1-乙基-7-氯-6-氟-1，4-二氢-4-氧代喹啉-3-羧酸乙酯（乙基物）制备

向装有搅拌器、回流冷凝器、温度计、滴液漏斗的 250 ml 四颈瓶中，加入环合物 25 g、无水碳酸钾 30.8 g、DMF 125 g，搅拌，加热至 70 ℃，于 70～80 ℃滴加溴乙烷 25 g，40～60 分钟滴加完毕，升温至 100～110 ℃，反应 6～8 小时，减压回收 70%～80%的 DMF，降温至 50 ℃左右，加入 200 ml 水，析出固体，过滤，水洗，干燥，得粗品，用乙醇重结晶，过滤，干燥，称重，计算产率。

注意事项

1. 反应所用 DMF 需预先干燥，水分对产率影响很大。

2. 溴乙烷沸点低，易挥发，为避免损失，可将滴液漏斗的滴管加长，插到液面以下，同时注意反应装置的密闭性。

3. 反应液加水时，温度要降至 50 ℃左右，过高，酯键易水解，过低，产物易结块，不易处理。

4. 环合物在溶液中酮式与烯醇式有一平衡，反应后可得到少量 O-乙基化合物，该化合物随主产物一起进入后续反应，生成 6-氟-1，4-二氢-4-氧代-7-（1-哌嗪基）喹

啉（简称脱羧物），成为诺氟沙星中的主要杂质。不同的乙基化试剂，O-乙基产物生成量不一样，采用 BrEt 时较低。

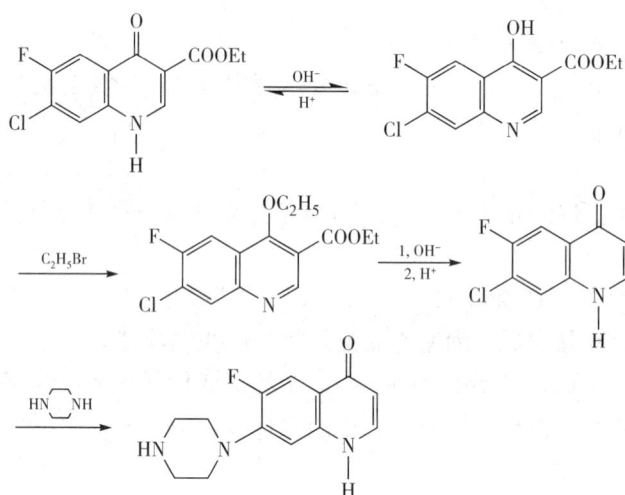

5. 滤饼洗涤时要将颗粒碾细，同时用大量水冲洗，否则会有少量 K_2CO_3 残留。

6. 乙醇重结晶操作过程：取粗品，加入 4 倍量的乙醇，加热至沸腾，溶解。稍冷，加入活性炭，回流 10 分钟，趁热过滤，滤液冷却至 10 ℃结晶析出，过滤，洗涤，干燥，得精品，测熔点（mp.144～145 ℃）。母液中尚有部分产品，可以浓缩一半体积后，冷却，析晶，所得产品亦可用于下步投料。

（七）1-乙基-7-氯-6-氟-1,4-二氢-4-氧代喹啉-3-羧酸（水解物）的制备

向装有搅拌器、回流冷凝器、温度计的三颈瓶中，加入乙基物 20 g 以及碱液（由氢氧化钠 5.5 g 和蒸馏水 75 g 配成），加热至 95～100 ℃，反应 10 分钟。冷却至 50 ℃，加水 125 ml 稀释，浓盐酸调 pH＝6，冷却至 20 ℃，过滤，水洗，干燥，称重，计算产率。测产物熔点（若熔点低于 270 ℃，需进行重结晶）。

注意事项

1. 由于反应物不溶于碱，而产品溶于碱，反应完全后，反应液澄清。

2. 在调 pH 之前应粗略计算盐酸用量，临近终点时，滴加稀盐酸，防止加入的酸过量。

3. 重结晶方法：取粗品，加入 5 倍量上步回收的 DMF，加热溶解，加入活性炭，再加热，过滤，除去活性炭，冷却，结晶，过滤，洗涤，干燥，得精品。

（八）诺氟沙星的制备

向装有搅拌器、回流冷凝器、温度计的 150 ml 三颈瓶中，加入水解物 10 g、无水哌嗪 13 g、吡啶 65 g，回流反应 6 h，冷却至 10 ℃，析出固体，抽滤，干燥，称重，测熔点，mp. 215～218 ℃。

将上述粗品加入 100 ml 水溶解，用冰醋酸调 pH＝7，抽滤，得精品，干燥，称重，计算该步产率和总产率。测终产物熔点（mp. 216～220 ℃）。

注意事项

反应物的 6 位氟亦可与 7 位氯竞争性地参与反应，会有氯哌酸副产物生成，最多可达 25%。

（九）硼螯合物的制备

向装有搅拌器、回流冷凝器、温度计、滴液漏斗的 250 ml 四颈瓶中，加入适量氯化锌、硼酸 3.3 g 及少量醋酐（醋酐总用量为 17 g），搅拌，加热至 79 ℃，反应引发后，停止加热，自动升温至 120 ℃。滴加剩余醋酐，滴加完毕后回流 1 小时，冷却，加入乙基物 10 g，回流 2.5 小时，冷却到室温，加水，过滤，少量冰乙醇洗至灰白色，干燥，称重，计算产率。测产物熔点（mp. 275 ℃，分解）。

注意事项

1. 硼酸与醋酐反应生成硼酸三乙酰酯，此反应到达 79 ℃临界点时才开始反应，并释放出大量热量，温度急剧升高。如果未反应物量大，则有冲料的危险，建议采用 250 ml 以上的反应瓶，并缓慢加热。

2. 由于螯合物在乙醇中有一定溶解度，为避免产品损失，最后洗涤时，可先用冰水洗涤，温度降下来后，再用冰乙醇洗涤。

（十）诺氟沙星的制备

向装有搅拌器、回流冷凝器、温度计的三颈瓶中，加入螯合物 10 g、无水哌嗪 8 g、二甲亚砜（DMSO）30 g，于 110 ℃反应 3 小时，冷却至 90 ℃，加入 10% NaOH 20 ml，回流 2 小时，冷至室温，加 50 ml 水稀释，用乙酸调 pH 7.2，过滤，水洗，得粗品。在 250 ml 烧杯中加入粗品及 100 ml 水，加热溶解后，冷却，用乙酸调 pH=7，析出固体，抽滤，水洗，干燥，称重，计算该步产率和总产率。测终产物熔点（mp. 216～220 ℃）。

注意事项

1. 硼螯合物可以利用 4 位羰基氧的 p 电子向硼原子轨道转移的特性，增强诱导效应，激活 7-Cl，钝化 6-F，从而选择性地提高哌嗪化产率，能彻底地防止氯哌酸的生成。

2. 由于诺氟沙星溶于碱，如反应液在加入 NaOH 回流后澄清，表示反应已进行完全。

3. 过滤粗品时，要将滤饼中的乙酸盐洗净，防止带入精制过程，影响产品质量。

五、思考

1. 配制混酸时能否将浓硝酸加到浓硫酸中？为什么？

2. 氟化反应产率提高的关键是什么？水溶液中的二甲亚砜如何回收？

3. 4-氟-3-氯-苯胺的制备中，如何检测反应的终点？反应中为何分步投料？

4. 1-乙基-7-氯-6-氟-1,4-二氢-4-氧代喹啉-3-羧酸（水解物）的制备中，浓盐酸调 pH 临近 6 时，溶液会有什么变化？

Experiment 9　Synthesis of Norfloxacin

1. Objective

1.1　To master the basic process of drug synthesis through the synthesis of norfloxacin.

1.2　To master the basic requirments for choosing actual production technique through the comparison of synthesis routes.

1.3　To master the quality controlling method of each reaction intermediate.

2. Principle

The chemical name of norfloxacin is 1-ethyl-6-fluoro-1,4-dihydro-4-oxo-7- (1-piperaznyl) - 3-quino-linecarboxylic acid. Its structure is as follows:

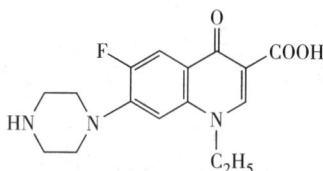

Norfloxacin is light yellow acicular or minute crystals, soluble in acid and base, hardly soluble in cool water.

According to the raw material and the synthetic routes, there are many metheds to prepare norfloxacin. The industrial production in our country primarily use route 1. In the last few years, many new techniques had been applied to synthesize norfloxacin, such as route 2. The method of boron chelated complex has a higher yield, simple operation, low loss and excellent quality.

The synthesis route is as follows:

Route 1

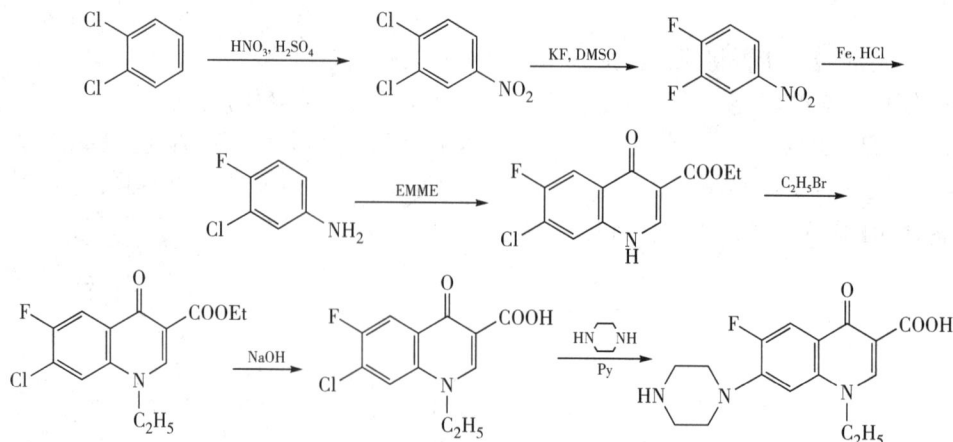

Route 2

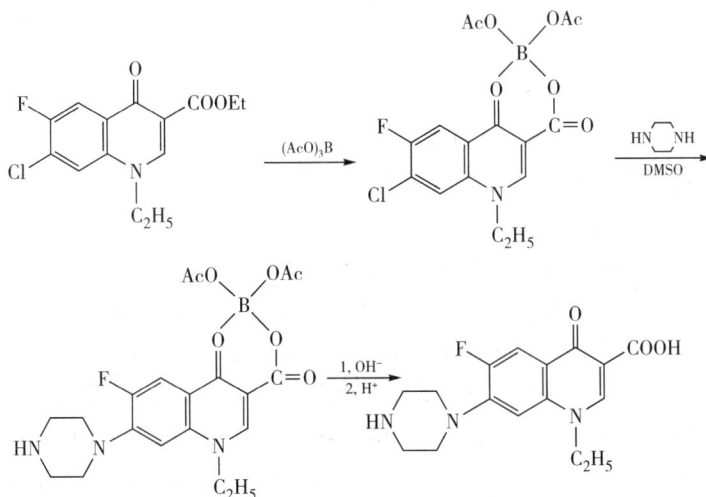

3. Apparatus and Materials

Apparatus: magnetic heating stirrer, condenser-Allihn type, thermometer, four-neck flask (250 ml), dropping funnel, round bottom flask (100 ml), beaker (250 ml), Busher funnel, suction flask.

Materials: nitric acid, concentrated sulfuric acid, 1,2-dichlorobenzene, 3,4-dichloride, DMSO, potassium fluoride, iron, sodium chloride, $ZnCl_2$, triethoxymethane, acetic anhydride, anhydrous potassium carbonate, DMF, anhydrous piperazine.

4. Procedures

4.1 Synthesis of 3, 4-dichloronitrobenzene

Nitric acid (51 g) was added into a four-neck flask equipped with an efficient mercury-sealed stirrer, a dropping funnel, a thermometer, and a reflux condenser. Sulfuric acid (79 g) was dropwise added, with water cooling to make sure that the temperature was below 50 ℃. Then, 1,2~dichlorobenzene (35 g) was also dropwise added about 40 min with the temperature at about 40~50 ℃. Following, the temperature was raised to 60 ℃ for 2 hours. The organic layer was carefully poured into water (5 times volume of the organic layer), stirred to form crystals about 30 min, filtered, washed with water until the pH of the filtrate was about 6~7, dried in vacuum, weighed, calculated yields.

Notes:

a. The nitration reacted with the nitro-sulfuric acid. And the sulfuric acid could prevent side reaction and increase the solubility of nitration product. NO_2^+ from nitric acid was the nitrating agent.

b. The temperature of this nitration must achieve 40 ℃. Below this temperature, dropwise adding nitro-sulfuric acid would cause accumulation of it, which would result in high temperature and produce much by-product or cause to explode. Therefore, dropwise adding nitro-sulfuric acid, the temperature should be at 40~50 ℃.

c. The product obtained from above method was pure enough for the next step. It also could be distilled with steam or reduced pressure to obtain purer product.

d. The melting point of 3,4-dicholoronitrobenzene is 39~41 ℃, therefore, it could not be dried with infra-red lamp or oven.

4.2 Synthesis of 4-fluoro-3-chloronitrobenzene

3,4-dichloride (40 g), DMSO (73 g) and potassium fluoride (23 g) were added into a four-neck flask with an efficient mercury-sealed stirrer, a thermometer, a reflux condenser and a calcium chloride drying tube. The mixture was refluxed at 194~198 ℃ for 1~1.5 hours, then cooled to 50 ℃, stirred completely after adding H_2O (75 ml). The mixture was separated into a separating funnel. The organic layer was refined by steam distillation obtained light yellow solid, which was washed until pH = 7, dried in vacuum, weighed, calculated yields.

Notes:

a. This reaction must be anhydrous absolutely including all instruments, reagents and drugs. A little water can make the yield decreased dramatically.

b. In order to render certain the anhydrous condition, a little of DMSO was distilled off to carry off the residuary water just before the reaction.

c. A little of condensed water was enough when distilled with steam. 4 - fluoro - 3 - chloronitrobenzene would be solidied and blocked the condenser when the condensed water was too much.

4.3 Synthesis of 4-fluoro-3-chloroaminobenzene

Iron (51.5 g), water (173 ml), sodium chloride (4.3 g) and concentrated hydrochloric acid (2.0 ml) were added into a three-necked flask with a stirrer, a thermometer and a reflux condenser. The mixture was stirred for 10 min at 100 ℃, added 15 g of the 4-fluoro-3-chloroaminobenzene (15 g) was added when the temperature drop to 85 ℃, then the temperature would raise to 95 ℃, the other 4-fluoro-3-chloroaminobenzene (15 g) was added after 10 min, And the mixture reacted for 2 hours at 95 ℃. The mixture was refined by steam distillation. The product was crystallized from the distillate after adding ice, filtered, dried in vacuum, weighed, calculated yields. (product, mp. 44~47 ℃)

Notes:

a. The amine is usually prepared by iron powder to reduce the nitro compounds when hydrochloric acid or acetic acid exists. Cheap materials, simple operation, stable yield and suitable for industrial production are the advantages of the method.

b. Because the iron powder has iron oxide film, it must be activated before hand. Generally, the granularity of the powdered iron is 60 item.

c. Because of the high density of iron dust, the stirring speed should be fierce. Otherwise it could not mix the iron dust evenly, further would agglomerate lower part of flask, influence the yield.

d. The flow rate of cooling water should be controlled during steam distillation in order to prevent 4-fluoro-3-chloroaniline to solidify and further jam condenser.

e. Melting point of 4-fluoro-3-chloroaniline is low (40~43 ℃), therefore it should be dried at low temperature.

4.4　Synthesis of EMME

Triethoxymethane (78 g) and ZnCl$_2$ (0.1 g) were added into a four-necked flask equipped with a stirrer, a dropping funnel, a thermometer and a reflux condenser. Elcohol was distilled at 120 ℃. Then the temperature was droped to 70 ℃, 20 g of triethoxymethane (20 g) and acetic anhydride (6.0 g) were dropwise added at 60~70 ℃. After that, the mixture was reacted at 152~156 ℃ for 2 hours, then, cooled to room temperature. The solution of reaction was carefully poured into a round-bottom flask, distilled under vacuum with water pump to recycle triethoxymethane (bp. 140 ℃, 70 ℃/5333 Pa). Lastly cooled to room temperature, the residue was distilled under reduced pressure with oil pump to collect fraction (120~140 ℃/666.6 Pa). weighed, calculated yields.

Notes:

a. The vacuum degree had to reach below 666.6 Pa, if not the yield would be very low.

b. The triethoxymethane could also be distilled at normal pressure, And the distillate was collected at 140－150 ℃. Thetriethoxymethane could be recycled.

4.5　Synthesis of 7-chloro-6-fluoro-1, 4-dihydro-4-oxo-quinoline-3-carboxylic acid ethyl ester (ring compound)

4-floro-3-chloroaniline (15.0 g) and EMME (24.0 g) were added into a three-necked flask with a sealed stirrer, a thermometer and a reflux condenser. The mixture was reacted at 120~130 ℃ for 2 h, cooled to r.t, added 80 ml paraffin oil, heated up to 260~270 ℃, distilled the alcohol, 30 minutes later, dropped the temperature to 60 ℃, filtered, washed with methylbenzene and acetone, dried in vacuum, weighed, calculated yields. (product, mp. 297~298 ℃)

Notes:

a. This reaction should be anhydrous include all instruments reagents and drugs., otherwise it could cause EMME to decompose.

b. The temperature of cyclization should be controlled at 260~270 ℃, gradually heated up when the temperature approached 270 ℃. The mixture became thick upon a time, therefore stirred fast in order to avoid partial heating.

c. The cyclization is a typical Could-Jacobs reaction. Because of orientation effect and steric effect of substitution on the benzene ring, para-position substitution of 3-chlorine is much more active than ortho-position substitution, but cannot aviod the ortho-position substitution. If the condition controls is improper, then the counter-link could be produced:

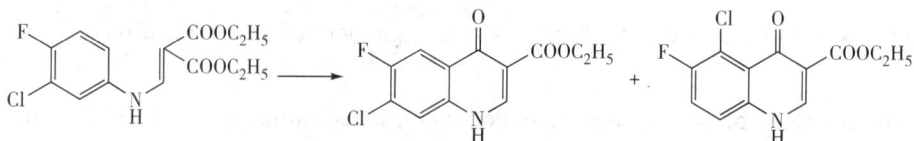

In order to reduce the counter-link product, the following several points should be paid attention to: (a) Low reaction temperature is favoured to obtain the counter-link product, therefore, the reaction temperature should quickly achieve 260 ℃, and maintain at 260～270 ℃. (b) Enlarging the amount of solvent may reduce the counter-link product. Moreover, according to economical factor, the solvent and the reactant amount (3/1) is more appropriate. (c) If xylene or benzion sulphone is used as solvent, the counter-link production could be reduced. Because the price of the solvent is high, we usually use the inexpensive industrial diesel oil to replace the paraffin oil.

4.6　Synthesis of 1-ethyl-7-chloro-6-fluoro-1,4-dihydro-4-oxo-quinoline-3-carboxylic acid ethyl ester (ethyl compound)

Cyclization (25.0 g), anhydrous potassium carbonate (30.8 g) and DMF (125 g) were added into a four-necked flask (250 ml) equipped with an efficient mercury-sealed stirrer, a dropping funnel, a thermometer and a reflux condenser. Ethyl bromide was dropwise added within 40～60 min at 70～80 ℃. Then,the mixture reacted for 6～8 h at 100～110 ℃. Distilled DMF, cooled to 50 ℃, following up, water (200 ml) was added into the organic layer. At last a mass of crystals formed, filtered, washed with water, dried, a raw product was obtained, crystallized with ethyl alcohol, filtered, washed, dried, weighed, calculated yields.

Notes:

a. DMF had to be dry in advance. A little of water would influence the yield seriously. And the anhydrous potassium carbonate needed to be fried.

b. The boiling point of ethyl bromide is low, and it is easy to volatilize. In order to avoid losing, the dropping funnel dropper, should be lengthened and set below the liquid level, meanwhile, the leakproofness should be paid more attention to.

c. The temperature was dropped to 50 ℃ by adding water. Because the ester bond is easy hydrolysis at high temperature. The product could cause to agglomerate at low temperature and was difficult to deal with.

d. There was a balance between ketonic and enol forms in the solution, might obtain a few ethyl compounds, which accompanied by the main product entering the next steps. At last 6-fluoro-4-oxo-7-piperazin-1-yl-1,4-dihydro-quinoline was produced, which was the main impurity. According to different ethylic reagent, the quantity of *O*-ethyl product is different. When the ethylic reagent is BrEt, the quantity of *O*-ethyl product is low relatively.

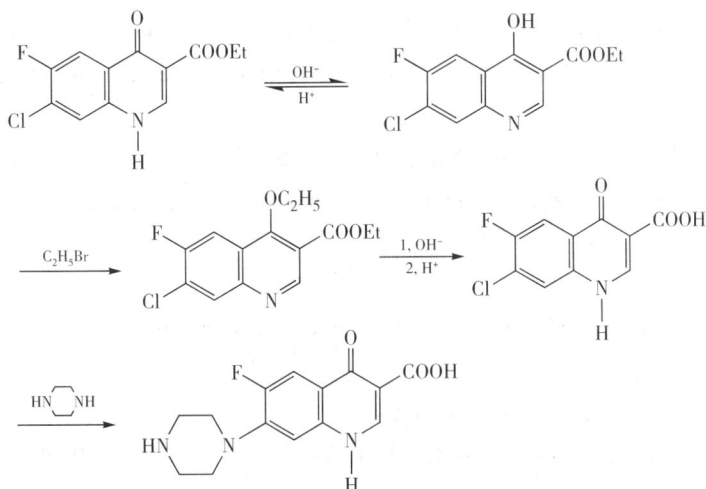

e. When washed the filter cake, the pellet should be made thin, at the same time massive water was used to flush, otherwise a few of K_2CO_3 would be remained.

f. The process of recrystallization with ethyl alcohol: Taked the crude product, added 4 times amount of ethyl alcohol, heated up to boil in order to dissolve. Slightly cool, the active charcoal was added, refluxed for 10 min, filtered when it was hot. cooled to 10 ℃ until crystallized. Filtered, washed, dried and obtained high-quality product, measured melting point (mp.144~145 ℃). Concentrated the mother liquor to a half-volume, cooled, the obtained product also could be used in the next step.

4.7　Synthesis of 1-ethyl-7-chloro-6-fluoro-1,4-dihydro-4-oxo-quinoline-3-carboxylic acid. (hydrolysate)

Ethide (20 g) and alkali solution (formed of 5.5 g NaOH and 75 g water) were added into a three-necked flask with a stirrer, a thermometer and a reflux condenser. The mixture was reacted at 95~100 ℃ for 10 min, cooled to 50 ℃, diluted with water (125 ml), adjusted the pH＝6 with HCl, dropped the temperature to 20 ℃, filtered, washed with water, dried, calculated the yield, measured the melting point (if below 270 ℃, recrystallization).

Notes:

a. Because the reactant did not dissolve in alkali solution, but the product dissolved in the alkali solution. The reaction fluid would be clear when finished.

b. Before adjusting pH, calculated the amount of hydrochloric acid firstly. When it is approximate to the end point, diluted hydrochloric acid was dropwise added avoid excessive acid.

c. The method of recrystallization: Take the crude product, 5 times the reclaimed DMF was added, heated up to dissolve and added the active charcoal, heated again, filtered the active charcoal off, cooled, filtered the crystallization, washed, dried and obtained high-quality product.

4.8　Synthesis of Norfloxacin

Hydrolysate (10.0 g), anhydrous piperazine (10.0 g) and pyridine (65 g) were added into a three-necked flask with a stirrer, a thermometer and a reflux condenser. The mixture was refluxed for 6 h, cooled to 10 ℃, then the solid was formed, filtered, dried, weighed, measured mp.(215～218 ℃)

The crude product was dissolved with 125 ml water. The pH was adjusted to 7 with glacial acetic acid, filtered, dried, weighed, calculated the yied of this step and the total yield, measured mp.(216～220 ℃)

Notes:

The reactant 6-fluoro might compete with 7-chloro, which produced by-product.The amount may reach 25% at most.

4.9　Synthesis of boron chelated complex

$ZnCl_2$, boric acid 3.3 g and a handful of acetic anhydride (total: 17 g) were added into a four-necked flask (250 ml) with a stirrer, a dropping funnel, a thermometer and a reflux condenser. The temperature was raised to 79 ℃. Once the reaction was started, stopped heating, the temperature would raise to 120 ℃ automatically. The other acetic anhydride was dropwise added, then, refluxed for 1 h. Cooled, ethide (10 g) was added, refluxed for 2.5 h, droped the temperature to r.t., added water, filtered, washed with ethyl alcohol till hoary, dried, calculated the yied, measured mp. 275 ℃ (decompose).

Notes:

a. The boric acid reacted with the acetic anhydride obtained triacetyl borate. When the temperature arrived at critical points (79 ℃), the reaction started and released a large amount of heat, Because the temperature raised suddenly, the mixture might flush. And it is suggested that the flask should be over 250 ml and heated up slowly.

b. Because the chelated complex dissolved in ethyl alcohol to some extent, in order to avoid loss, firstly washed with ice water, cooled down and washed with ethyl alcohol.

4.10　Synthesis of Norfloxacin

Chelated complex (10.0 g), anhydrous piperazine (8.0 g) and DMSO (30 g) were added into a three-necked flask with a stirrer, a thermometer and a reflux condenser. The mixture was allowed to stand at 110 ℃ for 3 h, cooled to 90 ℃, 10% NaOH (20 ml) was added, refluxed for 2 h, cooled to r.t, diluted with water (50 ml), it was adjusted to pH = 7.2 with acetic acid, filtered, washed with water to obtain the crude product. Placed the crude product and water (100 ml) in a beaker (250 ml), heated to dissolve, cooled. The pH was adjusted to 7 with acetic acid, solid was formed, filtered, washed with water, dried, calculated the yied of this step and the total yied, measured the end-product mp. (216～220 ℃).

Notes:

a. Boron chelated complex used the characteristic p electrons in 4−ketone oxygens, enhanced inductive effect, activated 7-Cl, deactivated 6-F, thus the yield was enhanced selectively, and norfloxacin would be produced thoroughly.

b. Norfloxacin can dissolve in alkali solution. If the reaction fluid turned to be clear after

NaOH was added, which indicated that the reaction was finished completely.

c. When filtered the crude product, the acetate should be washed out in the filter cake in order not to be brought into the process of purification.

5. Questions

5.1　Whether could the nitric acid be dropwise added into the sulfuric acid or not? Why?

5.2　What was the critical factor to improve the yied in fluoridation? How to recycle the DMSO in the aqueous solution?

5.3　How to examine the reaction endpoint in reaction of synthesis of 4-fluoro-3-chloroaminobenzene? Why should add the materials in step-by-step?

5.4　What would be happen to the solution when pH was adjusted to 6 with concentratedhydrochloric acid? Why?

实验十　苯妥英钠的合成

一、实验目的

1. 学习二苯羟乙酸重排反应原理。
2. 掌握用三氯化铁氧化的实验方法。

二、实验原理

苯妥英钠为抗癫痫药，适于治疗癫痫大发作，也可用于三叉神经痛及某些类型的心律失常的治疗。

化学名：5,5-二苯基-2,4-咪唑烷二酮钠盐，具环状酰脲结构。

化学结构式：

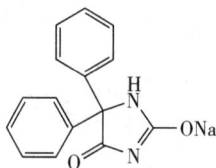

苯妥英钠为白色粉末，无臭、味苦。微有吸湿性，易溶于水，能溶于乙醇，几乎不溶于乙醚和三氯甲烷。mp. 222～227 ℃。

合成路线如下：

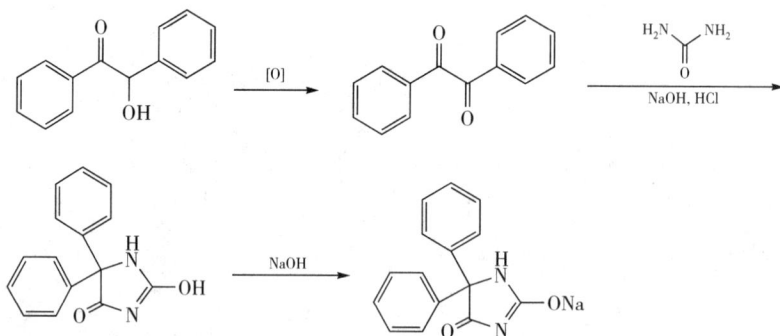

三、仪器和试剂

仪器：磁力加热搅拌器，球形冷凝器，温度计，三颈瓶（250 ml），圆底烧瓶（100 ml），烧杯（250 ml），布氏漏斗，抽滤瓶。

试剂：安息香，硝酸，$FeCl_3 \cdot 6H_2O$，冰醋酸，尿素，20% NaOH，50% 乙醇，10% 盐酸，活性炭。

四、实验步骤

（一）联苯甲酰的制备

方法 1：在装有搅拌子、温度计和球形冷凝管的 100 ml 三颈瓶中，加入安息香 6 g，硝酸（$HNO_3:H_2O=1:0.6$）15 ml，开动搅拌器，油浴加热，逐渐升温至 110～120 ℃，反应 2 小时（反应中产生的氧化氮气体，可从冷凝管顶端装一导管，将其通入水池中排出）。反应完毕，在搅拌下，将反应液倾入 40 ml 热水中，搅拌至结晶全部析出。抽滤，用少量冷水清洗结晶，干燥，得粗品。

方法 2：在装有搅拌子、温度计和球形冷凝管的 250 ml 圆底烧瓶中，依次加入 $FeCl_3 \cdot 6H_2O$ 21 g，冰醋酸 20 ml，水 10 ml，加热沸腾 5 分钟。稍冷，加入安息香 5 g，加热回流 50 分钟。稍冷，加水 80 ml，再加热至沸腾后，将反应液倾入 250 ml 烧杯中，搅拌，放冷，析出黄色固体，抽滤。用少量水清洗结晶，干燥，得粗品。测熔点，mp. 88～90 ℃，计算收率。

（二）苯妥英的制备

在装有搅拌子、冷凝管和温度计的 100 ml 三颈瓶中，依次加入联苯甲酰 4 g，尿素 1.4 g，20% NaOH 水溶液 12 ml，50% 乙醇 20 ml，开动搅拌器，油浴加热，回流反应 30 分钟。反应完毕，在搅拌下，将反应液倾入 120 ml 沸水中，加入适量活性炭，煮沸 5 分钟，放冷，抽滤。滤液用 10% 盐酸调至 pH 6，放置析出结晶。抽滤，用少量水清洗结晶，干燥，得苯妥英粗品。

（三）成盐与精制

将苯妥英粗品置 100 ml 烧杯中，按粗品与水为 1:4 的比例加入水，油浴加热至 40 ℃，加入 20% NaOH 至全溶，加活性炭少许，在搅拌下加热 5 分钟，趁热抽滤，滤液加氯化钠至饱和。放冷，析出结晶，抽滤，用少量冰水洗涤，干燥得苯妥英钠，称重，计算收率。

（四）结构确证

1. 红外吸收光谱、标准物 TLC 对照法。
2. 核磁共振光谱法。

五、注意事项

1. 硝酸为强氧化剂，使用时应避免与皮肤、衣服等接触，氧化过程中，硝酸被还原产生氧化氮气体，该气体具有一定刺激性，须控制反应温度，以防止反应激烈，大量氧化氮气体逸出。

2. 制备钠盐时，水量稍多，可使收率受到明显影响，要严格按比例加水。

六、思考

1. 制备联苯甲酰时，反应温度为什么要逐渐升高？氧化剂为什么不用硝酸，而用稀硝酸？
2. 本品精制的原理是什么？

Experiment 10   Synthesis of Phenytoin Sodium

1. Objective

1.1   To study the rearrangement mechanism of benzilic acid.
1.2   To master the experiment method of oxidation with $FeCl_3$.

2. Principle

Phenytoin Sodium can be used as an antiepileptic for treatment with grand mal epilepsy and for trifacial neuralgia or for some arrhythmia. The chemical name of phenytoin sodium is 5, 5-diphenylhydantoin sodium, and its chemical structure is as following:

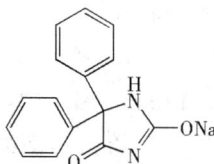

Phenytoin sodium is a white powder, odorless, bitter in taste, slightly hygroscopic, mp. $222 \sim 227 \ ℃$, and is soluble in water and ethanol, but almost insoluble in chloroform and ether.

The synthetic route is as following:

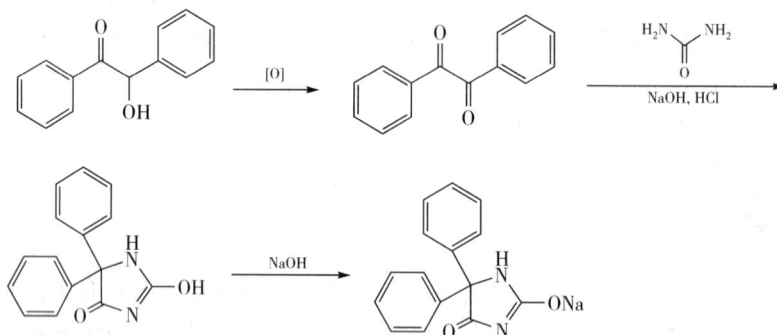

3. Apparatus and Materials

Apparatus: magnetic heating stirrer, condenser-Allihn type, thermometer, three necked flask（250 ml）, round bottom flask（100 ml）, beaker（250 ml）, Busher funnel, suction flask.

Materials: benzoin, nitric acid, $FeCl_3 \cdot 6H_2O$, active carbon, dibenzoyl, urea, 20% NaOH, 50% ethanol, sodium chloride.

4. Procedures

4.1 Synthesis of dibenzoyl

Method A: In a 100 ml round bottom flask equipped with stirrer, thermometer and a round condenser, benzoin 6 g and nitric acid（HNO_3:H_2O = 1:0.6）15 ml was added. Stirred the reaction mixture, heated to 110~120 ℃ for 2 h in oil bath (the NO gas produced in the reaction was discharged to a water pool through a canula equipped onto the top of condenser). When the reaction was completed, the reaction mixture was poured into 40 ml of hot water with stirring till the crystal precipitated completely. The solid precipitate was collected by vacuum filtration and washed with a small amount of cold water, dried and the crude product was obtained.

Method B: In a 250 ml round bottom bottle equipped with stirrer, thermometer and a round condenser, $FeCl_3 \cdot 6H_2O$ 21 g, 20 ml of ice acetic acid and water 10 ml were added, heated to reflux for 5 min on oil bath. After cooling for a while, added benzoin 5 g, and then heated to reflux for 50 min. Then added another 80 ml of water and heated to reflux again. When the reaction was completed, poured the mixture into a 250 ml beaker. Stirred and cooled thoroughly, then separated out the yellow solid by vacuum filtration. Washed the crystal with a small amount of cold water, dried and the crude product was obtained. Measured the melting point, mp. 88~90 ℃, and calculate the yield.

4.2 Synthesis of Phenytoin

In a 100 ml round bottom bottle equipped with a condenser, dibenzoyl 4 g, urea 1.4 g, 20% NaOH 12 ml and 50% ethanol 20 ml were added, stirred and heated to reflux for 30 mins. The reaction mixture was poured into 120 ml of hot water after the reaction accomplished, then added active carbon and boiled for 5 min. Cooled and filtrated it. Adjusted the filtration to pH 6 with 10% HCl solution, placed and then separated out the crystal by vacuum filtration, washed with a small amount of water, dried and the crude phenytoin was obtained.

4.3 Salification and refinement

The crude phenytoin was added into a 100 ml beaker, added 4 folds of water, heated to 40 ℃ in a water bath, and added 20% NaOH till the solid dissolved completely. Added a little active carbon, heated for 5 min under stirring, filtrated while heating, and then added sodium chloride (NaCl) into the filtration until saturation. Cooled, separated the crystal, filtrate, washed with a small amount of icy-water. Dried and phenytoin sodium was obtained. Weighed and calculate the yield.

4.4 Identification

4.4.1 Infrared absorption spectroscopy, TLC confrontation experiment with standard substance.

4.4.2 Nuclear magnetic resonance spectroscopy.

5. Notes

5.1 Nitric acid is a strong oxidant which should not be contacted with skin, clothes and other things. Nitric acid will be reduced and produced NO (a gas) which has a certainty thrill in the course of oxidation, so the reaction temperature should be controlled in order to prevent the reaction too severely and transgress too much NO gas.

5.2   A little excessively water will obviously affect the yield in the preparation of the sodium salt, so the water should be added strictly.

6. Questions

6.1   Why should reaction temperature rise gradually during the preparation of benzoin? Why not use nitric acid but dilute nitric acid as oxidizer?

6.2   What is the principle of the Phenytoin Sodium's refinement?

实验十一 TLC（薄层层析色谱）技术原理与应用

一、实验目的

1. 通过实验加深对薄层色谱法原理的理解。
2. 掌握薄层色谱法分离、鉴定药物的操作技术。

二、实验原理

薄层层析是一种简便、快速的分离分析方法，广泛应用于纯物质的鉴定和混合物的分离、提纯及含量的测定，也常用作摸索和确定柱层析的洗脱条件。

薄层层析是指吸附剂铺成的薄层所进行的层析，吸附薄层中常用的吸附剂为氧化铝和硅胶等。其原理主要是利用吸附剂（固定相）对样品中各成分吸附能力不同，及展开剂（流动相）对它们的解吸附能力的不同，使各成分达到分离。

薄层层析过程中，在展开剂的作用下，样品中的混合组分在展开剂和薄层板之间不断地产生吸附、解吸、再吸附、再解吸的反复过程。吸附强度取决于吸附剂的吸附能力，同时还受被吸附成分本身性质的影响，更与展开剂的性质有关。展开剂通常是由两种或者两种以上的溶剂按照一定的比例组成的混合溶剂系统。用极性适当的展开剂浸润已经点了样品的薄层板一端，凭借毛细作用带动样品在薄层板上移动，最终使样品中不同的组分分离的操作过程。

化合物在吸附薄层上移动的速度与展开剂的极性有关。展开剂的极性越大，化合物移动的速度越快，反之，移动速度就越慢。待分离组分的极性决定于其母核结构类型及官能团的极性。在吸附剂活性和展开剂活性固定不变的条件下，待分离组分的极性越大，吸附剂对其吸附作用越强，展开距离越短；待分离组分极性越弱，吸附剂对其作用越大，展开距离越大。

展开结束后，经过显色操作，样品中各个成分会被分离并形成不同位移的斑点，为了表达各成分的相对位置（极性）通常以比移值作为称量斑点位置的指标。比移值的符号为 R_f：

R_f=(斑点中心与原始样点之间的距离)/(溶剂前沿与原始样点之间的距离)。

图 11-1 中化合物 A 的 R_f=a/c，化合物 B 的 R_f=b/c。

R_f 值的最佳范围在 0.3~0.7。如果 R_f 较大可适量加入极性较小的溶剂，以降低展开剂极性；反之，加入极性大的溶剂。根据分离化合物的结构、固定相与流动相的性质、温度等因素的不同而变化。当实验条件固定时，R_f 值为一个特定的常数，可以作为定性分析的依据。但是由于影响 R_f 值的因素较多，实

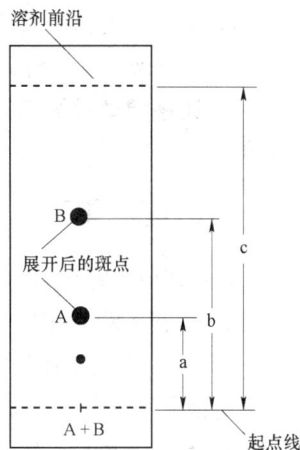

图 11-1 TLC 示意图

验数据通常与文献记载不完全相同，因此在药物鉴定时常用标准样品作对照分析。

三、仪器和试剂

仪器：层析缸，玻璃板（1.5 cm×100 cm），毛细管，喷雾器，电吹风，尺子，台秤，烘箱，量筒。

药品：硅胶 G，0.1% 羧甲基纤维素钠，0.1 g/L 胆固醇二氯甲烷溶液，0.1 g/L 可的松二氯甲烷溶液，待分离溶液（0.1 g/L 胆固醇与 0.1 g/L 可的松二氯甲烷混合溶液），展开剂（石油醚∶乙酸乙酯＝2∶1），20% 硫酸乙醇溶液。

四、实验步骤

1. 制备薄板　取两块玻璃板，洗净晾干，备用。称取 4 g 硅胶 G 置于小烧杯内，加 0.1% 羧甲基纤维素钠 10 ml，搅拌调成均匀的糊状，用吸管或玻璃棒在玻璃板上快速涂抹均匀，可以用拇指和食指拿住玻璃板做前后左右摇晃摆动，使流动的硅胶混悬液均匀地平铺在玻璃板上，也可将玻璃板在台面上轻轻跌落数次（附注 1）。然后将玻璃板置于水平台面上，室温晾半小时，放入烘箱内缓慢升温至 110 ℃，加热活化半小时，放冷后，置于干燥器中备用。

2. 点样　将样品溶于展开剂极性相近、挥发性高的有机溶剂。在薄层板一端距离底边 1 cm 处，用铅笔轻轻划一直线，作为点样线。用管口平整的毛细管（0.5 mm 以下）点加样品（附注 2）。样品斑点的扩散直径尽量小，以小于 2～3 mm 为宜；若一次点样浓度不够时，可在溶剂挥发后间隔反复点样；多个样品点时，各样点之间的距离应间隔为 1 cm 左右，且处于同一条直线上。

3. 展开　向洁净的层析缸内加入展开剂 30 ml，加盖密闭使溶剂蒸气饱和 5～10 分钟。再将已点样品的薄板水平放入层析缸内，点样一端朝下，浸入展开剂约 0.5 cm，注意勿使样品浸入展开剂，密闭层析缸。当展开剂前沿上升处距薄板上端约 1.0 cm 处时，取出薄板，用铅笔快速在展开剂上升的前沿处划一记号（附注 3）。晾干，也可用电吹风从硅胶板反面吹干。

4. 显色　将薄板均匀地喷上 20% 硫酸乙醇溶液，在 105 ℃加热 10 分钟后，放冷置紫外灯（365 nm）下检视。

5. 比移值的计算与定性、定量　测量原点中心到斑点中心的距离，分别计算样品点的 R_f 值。

五、注意事项

1. 薄板制备好后，要求表面平滑均匀。否则，色谱分离结果不好。

2. 样点不能泡在展开剂中，薄层板浸入时不能歪斜进入。

3. 点样时，所用毛细管应专用，垂直点样，且使毛细管刚好接触薄层即可，切勿用力过重而使薄层表面破坏。

4. 展开结束后，应及时在溶剂前沿划上记号，否则展开剂挥发后，就无法确定展开剂上升的高度，即 c 值。

六、思考

1. 为什么在某些药物合成过程中，可以用薄层色谱法跟踪监测反应进度？
2. 层析缸内展开剂高度超过了点样线，对薄层色谱有何影响？

Experiment 11　Thin Layer Chromatography (TLC)

1. Objective

1.1　To understand the principle of TLC.

1.2　To grasp the basic technique of TLC operation and its application in drug synthesis and drug identification.

2. Principle

Chromatography is a term applied to several separation techniques bases on differential migration. It makes use heterogeneous equilibrium established during the flow of a solvent called the mobile phase through a fixed (stationary) phase to separate two or more components from material carried by the solvent. Chromatography can be classified as adsorption chromatography, distribution chromatography and ion-exchange chromatography based on different relationship of substance between the two phases of the system in use. Basing on the different support of operation it can be named as: thin layer chromatography (TLC), paper chromatography (PC), and column chromatography (CC).

Thin layer chromatography is a sensitive, fast, simple, and inexpensive analytical technique that will be used repeatedly in carrying out organic experiments. It is a true micro technique; as little as 10^{-9} g of material can be detected.

TLC involves spotting the sample to be analyzed near one end of a sheet of glass, plastic, or aluminum coated with a thin layer of an adsorbent. The sheet which can be the size of a microscope slide, is placed on ended in a covered jar containing a shallow layer of solvent. As the solvent rises by capillary action up through the adsorbent, differential partitioning occurs between the components of the mixture dissolved in the solvent and the stationary adsorbent phase. The more strongly a given component of the mixture is adsorbed onto the stationary phase, the less time it will spend in the mobile phase and the more slowly it will migrate up the TLC plate.

The two most common coatings for thin-layer chromatography plates are alumina Al_2O_3, and silica, SiO_2. Of the two, alumina, when anhydrous, is the more active when the separation involves relatively nonpolar substrates. To separate the more polar substrates, silica gel, is used. A polar solvent will carry along with it polar substrates, and nonpolar solvent will do the same with nonpolar compounds another example of the generalization "like dissolves like".

The R_f value of the ratio of the distance the spot travels from the point of origin to the distance the travels (Fig. 11 − 1).The best separations are achieved when the R_f value falls between 0.3 and 0.7 without units.

$$R_f = \frac{\text{distance of center of the spot from the baseline (cm)}}{\text{distance of solvent from the baseline (cm)}}$$

R_f value of compound A is a/c, R_f value of compound B is b/c.

Where a, b – distance of center of the spot from the baseline. c – distance of solvent front from baseline.

It indicates that sample cannot mobile if R_f value is zero. The more different of R_f value between species of sample is, the better separation of mixture is.

3. Apparatus and Materials

Apparatus: glass plate (1.5 cm × 10 cm), medicine dropper, TLC tank mortar and pestle, oven, capillary tube, sprayer, graduated cylinder (10 ml), ruler, platform balance.

Materials: silica Gel G, 0.1 g/L cholesterol in dichloromethane, 0.1 g/L cortisone acetate in dichloromethane, 20% sulfuric acid in ethanol, developing solvent (petroleum ether:ethyl acetate = 2:1, v/v).

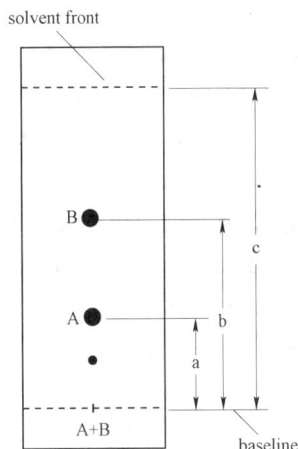

Fig: 11 – 1　TLC sketch

4. Procedures

4.1　Coating plates

The aqueous slurry（Note 1）of silica gel G is prepared by mixing about 3 g powder with 8 ml distilled water in mortal with pestle. Allow the plates to air dry at room temperature in the horizontal position, when the surface of the slides has become dull, then active them in an oven at 110 ℃ for 30 min before using.

4.2　Sample application

Following the procedure outline above, draw a light pencil line about 1 cm from the end of some chromatographic plates and on this line spot cholesterol, cortisone acetate, and their mixture (Note 2). Make each spot as small as possible, preferably less than 0.5 mm in diameter. If it is necessary to apply a larger amount (Note 3), let the first spot dry completely and then touch the capillary again at the same place. You should take care to make sure that each of the spots is the same distance from the bottom of the plate.

4.3　Elution

Pour 10 ml developing solvent of mixed benzene-ethyl acetate into the tank. Place the plate upright in the developing tank so that the sample end is immersed in the developing solvent to a depth of 0.5 cm. Do not put the spot immersed in the surface of solvent; the solvent should be introduced into the tank at least 15 minutes before commencing the separation. Allow the solvent to creep up the TLC plate until it is about 1.0 cm from the top. The plate is then removed from the developing tank, and mark（Note 4） the solvent front immediately with a small scratch. The solvent allowed to evaporate.

4.4 Visualization

The position of the separated solutes can be located by spraying the plate with a visualization reagent, which produces colored areas in the regions which samples occupy. In this case, 20% sulfuric acid in ethanol can be sprayed the plates after solvent evaporating completely. Put it in an oven at 110 ℃ for 10 minutes until the spots show.

4.5 Determination of R_f Value

Remove the chromatogram plate from the oven, and cool it room temperature. Circle each spot, and measure the distance from the origin to the center of each spot as well as the distance from the origin to the solvent front with ruler. Calculate all R_f values for any spots that are visible, and determine the identity of the unknown components. Record the chromatogram diagram in your report.

5. Notes

5.1 The object in plate coating is to spread a smooth, uniform layer that dries without bubbles, pits, or cracks.

5.2 You should make capillary tube just contact with a layer, rather than heavy spot, so as to avoid destroying the layer when the samples are applied.

5.3 The amount of each sample should be suitable. Overloaded sample applications produce comet-like vertical streaks or overlap on the chromatogram, while insufficient sample give poor separation which spots of some components can not appear.

5.4 The solvent front should be marked immediately after taking the layer out of TLC tank. Otherwise, you can not determinate the location of solvent after it evaporate.

6. Questions

6.1 Why in some drug synthesis, thin-layer chromatography can be used to monitor the extent of reaction?

6.2 What is the effect on thin layer chromatography if the spot is immersed in the surface of the solvent?

第三部分　附　录

附录一　旋转蒸发仪的使用

旋转蒸发仪主要用于在减压条件下连续蒸馏大量易挥发性溶剂。尤其对萃取液的浓缩和色谱分离时的接收液的蒸馏，可以分离和纯化反应产物。旋转蒸发仪的基本原理就是减压蒸馏，也就是在减压情况下，蒸馏烧瓶连续转动以增大蒸发面积，同时置于水浴锅中恒温加热，快速蒸馏溶剂。

一、结构

1. 具有操作简便的自动上下升降装置，手触上升键主机上升，手触下降键主机下降，手离键即停，操作方便。另备有应急手轮，当升降电机发生故障时，将手轮转动，主机也能上升或下降。

2. 独特密封结构和精选的密封材料，真空性能良好。

3. 温度由数字显示，控制由金属探头传感器来实现，当传感器插入加热槽（水浴锅）内，水温达到设定温度时会自动切断加热器电源，当水温低于设定选温度时会自动接通加热电源，如此交替来控制水温，可保持恒温。温控表拨位开关百位数必须置"O"位。

4. 加热槽选用优质不锈钢制成，为 220 mm×120 mm 的水浴锅，加热功率为 1.5kW，封闭式电阻加热器，锅内可装 2 L 烧瓶旋转。

5. 具有高蒸发率的立式冷凝器系统，内壁冷却水管由蛇行双回路玻璃管制成。当烧瓶旋转时，溶液在内壁扩散蒸发，然后通过大孔径蒸发管进入粗直径冷凝管加快蒸发。

二、安装

1. 安装时首先要调整机头角度，只要松开机头右边锁紧扳手即可调整，一般向右下倾斜 30°左右。调节时另一只手必须托住机头，调节后必须锁紧。然后支撑固定板装在机头左侧（出厂时已装好），螺钉暂不要拧紧。

2. 主轴安装：各个磨口接口及密封面、密封圈必须擦干净，安装前均需要涂一层真空脂，以防漏气，将螺母先套在主轴上，再把压紧圈套入主轴沉割槽处（必须嵌入凹槽内），然后扦入主轴旋转套内拧上螺母再用小六角扳手扦入机头下面小孔中寻找沉孔位再拧紧（在寻找时用另一只手转动螺母，让扳手对准沉孔位再拧紧，使主轴锁住，反之则可拆下主轴）。

3. 四通瓶的安装：将大塑料螺母先套入四通瓶颈，再把弹簧环也套进瓶颈，使卡牢瓶颈放在一边，然后按安装图把密封圈座套在主轴上，四氟圈座套在主轴上，最后把四通瓶上的大螺母拧入机头。

4. 冷凝瓶的安装：先套上不锈钢支撑夹圈，把冷凝瓶扦入四通瓶口上，并转动一下使接口接触紧密，此时套入竖杆中，调整位置后将螺丝拧紧。上端口装抽真空接头。

5. 加料管与放气开关出厂时已经装在一起，转动手柄 90 度能起到关闭或开通作用。最后安装蒸发器瓶和收液瓶，并用夹子夹紧。

三、使用方法

1. 高低调节：手动升降，转动机柱上面手轮，顺转为上升，逆转为下降。电动升降，手触上升键主机上升，手触下降键主机下降。

2. 冷凝器上有两个外接头是接冷却水用的，一头接进水，另一头接出水，一般接自来水，冷凝水温度越低效果越好。上端口装抽真空接头，接真空泵皮管抽真空用的。

3. 开机前先将调速旋钮左旋到最小，按下电源开关指示灯亮，然后慢慢往右旋至所需要的转速，一般大蒸发瓶用中、低速，黏度大的溶液用较低转速。烧瓶是标准接口 24 号，随机附 500、1000 ml 两种烧瓶，溶液量一般以不超过 50% 为适宜。

四、注意事项

1. 玻璃零件接装应轻拿轻放，装前应洗干净，擦干或烘干。

2. 各磨口、密封面密封圈及接头安装前都需要涂一层真空脂。

3. 加热槽通电前必须加水，不允许无水干烧。

4. 当体系与大气相通时，可以将蒸馏烧瓶、接液烧瓶取下，转移溶剂；当体系与减压泵相通时，则体系应处于减压状态。使用时，应先减压，再开动电动机转动蒸馏烧瓶。结束时，应先停机，再通大气，以防蒸馏烧瓶在转动中脱落。

5. 如真空抽不上来需检查：①各接头，接口是否密封。②密封圈，密封面是否有效。③主轴与密封圈之间真空脂是否涂好。④真空泵及其皮管是否漏气。⑤玻璃件是否有裂缝、碎裂、损坏的现象。

附录二 常见元素的原子量表

元素	符号	原子量	元素	符号	原子量	元素	符号	原子量
氢	H	1.007	氯	Cl	35.453	氪	Kr	83.798
氦	He	4.002	氩	Ar	39.948	铷	Rb	85.467
锂	Li	6.941	钾	K	39.098	锶	Sr	87.62
铍	Be	9.012	钙	Ca	40.078	钌	Ru	101.07
硼	B	10.811	钛	Ti	47.867	铑	Rh	102.905
碳	C	12.017	钒	V	50.941	钯	Pd	106.42
氮	N	14.006	铬	Cr	51.996	银	Ag	107.868
氧	O	15.999	锰	Mn	54.938	锡	Sn	118.710
氟	F	18.998	铁	Fe	55.845	碘	I	126.904
氖	Ne	20.179	钴	Co	58.933	铯	Cs	132.905
钠	Na	22.989	镍	Ni	58.693	钡	Ba	137.327
镁	Mg	24.305	铜	Cu	63.546	铂	Pt	195.084
铝	Al	26.981	锌	Zn	65.409	金	Au	196.966
硅	Si	28.085	砷	As	74.921	汞	Hg	200.59
磷	P	30.973	硒	Se	78.96	铅	Pb	207.2
硫	S	32.065	溴	Br	79.904	铋	Bi	208.980

附录三　常用的冰盐冷却剂

盐	每 100 g 碎冰用盐（g）	可降至温度（℃）
$NaNO_3$	50	−18.5
$NaCl$	33	−21.2
$NaCl$ NH_4Cl 混合物	40 20	−26
NH_4Cl $NaNO_3$ 混合物	13 37.5	−30.7
K_2CO_3	33	−46
$CaCl_2 \cdot H_2O$	143	−35

附录四 共沸混合溶剂

序号	溶剂	%（重量比）	沸点 770 mmHg	介电常数 ±0.0525 ℃
1	乙酸乙酯 环己烷	46.0 54.0	71.6	3.95
2	异丙醇 二异丙醚	16.3 83.7	66.2	5.75
3	乙醇 诺氯沙星	8.0 92.0	59.4	6.05
4	甲醇 诺氯沙星	12.6 87.4	53.4	9.80
5	甲醇 二氯甲烷	7.3 92.7	37.8	10.50
6	甲醇 乙酸乙酯	17.7 82.3	53.9	10.75
7	丙酮 环己烷	67.5 32.5	58.0	13.75
8	乙醇 甲苯	68.0 32.0	76.5	17.25
9	甲醇 丙酮	12.0 88.0	56.4	22.05
10	水 乙醇	4.0 96.0	78.2	25.40
11	甲醇 乙酸乙酯 三氯甲烷	21.6 27.0 51.4	56.4	13.65
12	乙醇 丙酮 三氯甲烷	10.4 24.3 65.3	63.2	13.90
13	甲醇 丙酮 三氯甲烷	23.0 30.0 47.0	57.5	19.30

附录五　常用有机溶剂的物理常数

溶剂	沸点（℃）	熔点（℃）	分子量	密度	介电常数	溶解度（g/100g 水）
乙醚	35	−116	74	.0.71	4.3	6.0
二硫化碳	46	−111	76	1.26	2.6	0.29（20℃）
丙酮	56	−95	58	0.79	20.7	∞
三氯甲烷	61.2	−64	119	1.49	4.8	0.82
甲醇	65	−98	32	0.79	32.7	∞
四氯化碳	77	−23	154	1.59	2.2	0.08
乙酸乙酯	77.1	−84	88	0.90	6.0	8.1
乙醇	78.3	−114	46	0.79	24.6	∞
苯	80.4	5.5	78	0.88	2.3	0.18
异丙醇	82.4	−88	60	0.79	19.9	∞
正丁醇	118	−89	74	0.81	17.5	7.45
甲酸	101	8	46	1.22	58.5	∞
甲苯	111	−95	92	0.87	2.4	0.05
吡啶	115	−42	79	0.98	12.4	∞
乙酸	118	17	60	1.05	6.2	∞
乙酸酐	140	−73	102	1.08	20.7	反应
硝基苯	211	6	123	1.20	34.8	0.19

附录六　常用的无机干燥剂

为了保持药品的干燥或对制得的气体进行干燥，必须使用干燥剂。常用的干燥剂有三类：一类为酸性干燥剂，有浓 H_2SO_4、五氧化二磷、硅胶等；第二类为碱性干燥剂，有固体烧碱、石灰和碱石灰（氢氧化钠和氧化钙的混合物）等；第三类是中性干燥剂，如无水氯化钙、无水硫酸镁等。

1. 浓 H_2SO_4　具有强烈的吸水性，常用来除去不与 H_2SO_4 反应的气体中的水分。例如常作为 H_2、O_2、CO、SO_2、N_2、HCl、CH_4、CO_2、Cl_2 等气体的干燥剂。

2. 无水氯化钙　因其价廉、干燥能力强而被广泛应用。干燥速度快，能再生，脱水温度 200 ℃。一般用以填充干燥器和干燥塔，干燥药品和多种气体。不能用来干燥氨、乙醇、胺、酰、酮、醛、酯等。

3. 无水硫酸镁　有很强的干燥能力，吸水后生成 $MgSO_4 \cdot 7H_2O$。吸水作用迅速，效率高，价廉，为一良好干燥剂。常用来干燥有机试剂。

4. 固体氢氧化钠和碱石灰　吸水快、效率高、价格便宜，是极佳的干燥剂，但不能用以干燥酸性物质。常用来干燥氢气、氧气和甲烷等气体。

5. 变色硅胶　常用来保持仪器、天平的干燥。吸水后变红。失效的硅胶可以经烘干再生后继续使用。可干燥胺、NH_3、O_2、N_2 等

6. 活性氧化铝（Al_2O_3）　吸水量大、干燥速度快，能再生（400～500 K 烘烤）。

7. 无水硫酸钠　干燥温度必须控制在 30 ℃ 以内，干燥性比无水硫酸镁差。

8. 硫酸钙　可以干燥 H_2、O_2、CO_2、CO、N_2、Cl_2、HCl、H_2S、NH_3、CH_4 等。

9. 分子筛干燥剂　它是人工合成且对水分子有较强吸附性的干燥剂产品。分子筛的孔径大小可通过加工工艺的不同来控制，除了吸附水气，它还可以吸附其他气体。在 230 ℃ 以上的高温情况下，仍能很好地容纳水分子。优点：适应性强。缺点：吸湿率低，环保差（不可降解）。

注：无水硫酸铜（$CuSO_4$）（无水硫酸铜为白色）也具有一定的干燥性，并且吸水后变成蓝色的五水硫酸铜（$CuSO_4 \cdot 5H_2O$），但一般不用来做干燥剂。

参考文献

［1］尤启东，王亚楼，李志裕，等. 药物化学实验与指导［M］. 北京：中国医药科技出版社，2000.

［2］李柱来，孟繁浩. 药物化学实验指导［M］. 北京：中国医药科技出版社，2016.

［3］闻韧. 药物合成反应［M］. 3版. 北京：化学工业出版社，2010.

［4］孙铁民. 药物化学实验［M］. 2版. 北京：中国医药科技出版社，2014.

［5］徐萍. 药物化学实验教程［M］. 北京：北京大学出版社，2010.

［6］吴珊珊. 相转移催化法合成扁桃酸的工艺研究［D］. 南京：南京理工大学硕士论文，2003.

［7］李公春，吴长增，郭俊伟. 苯妥英钠的合成［J］. 浙江化工，2015，46（8）：23.

［8］刘太泽. 苯佐卡因的合成研究［D］. 南昌：南昌大学硕士论文，2010.

［9］刘金，韦琨，蔡乐，等. 苯佐卡因的改进合成——推荐一个环保的多步合成实验［J］. 大学化学，2016，31（3）：64.

［10］熊海维，盐酸氯普鲁卡因的化学合成研究［D］. 杭州：浙江工业大学硕士论文，2009.